The Natural Medicine Guide to

AUTISM

Also by Stephanie Marohn

Natural Medicine First Aid Remedies

THE HEALTHY MIND GUIDES

The Natural Medicine Guide to AUTISM

Stephanie Marohn

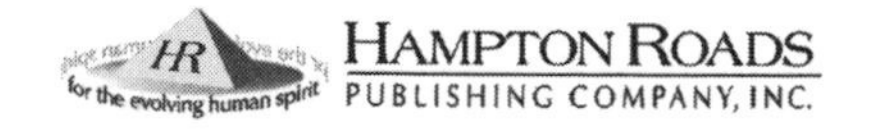

Cover design by Bookwrights Design
Cover art by Loyd Chapplow

Hampton Roads Publishing Company, Inc.
1125 Stoney Ridge Road
Charlottesville, VA 22902

434-296-2772
fax: 434-296-5096
e-mail: hrpc@hrpub.com
www.hrpub.com

If you are unable to order this book from your local
bookseller, you may order directly from the publisher.
Call 1-800-766-8009, toll-free.

Library of Congress Cataloging-in-Publication Data

Marohn, Stephanie.
The natural medicine guide to autism / Stephanie Marohn.
p. ; cm. -- (The healthy mind guides)
Includes bibliographical references and index.
ISBN 1-57174-288-3 (alk. paper)
1. Autism. 2. Autism--Alternative treatment. 3. Autistic
children--Alternative treatment. 4. Naturopathy.
[DNLM: 1. Autistic Disorder--Popular Works. 2. Naturopathy--
Popular Works. WM 203.5 M354n 2002] I. Title. II. Series.
RJ506.A9 M374 2002
618.92'898206--dc21

2002007637

ISBN 1-57174-288-3
10 9 8 7 6 5 4 3
Printed on acid-free paper in Canada

THE HEALTHY MIND GUIDES

THE HEALTHY MIND Guides is a series of books offering original research and treatment options for reversing or ameliorating several so-called mental disorders, written by noted health journalist and author Stephanie Marohn. The series' focus is the natural medicine approach, a refreshing and hopeful outlook based on treating individual needs rather than medical labels, and addressing the underlying imbalances—biological, psychological, emotional, and spiritual.

Each book in the series offers the very latest information about the possible causes of each disorder, and presents a wide range of effective, practical therapies drawn from extensive interviews with physicians and other practitioners who are innovators in their respective fields. Case studies throughout the books illustrate the applications of these therapies, and numerous resources are provided for readers who want to seek treatment.

The information in this book is not intended to replace medical care. The author and publisher disclaim responsibility for how you choose to employ the information in this book and the results or consequences of any of the treatments covered.

To all those who are facing the challenge of autism

Contents

Foreword

By Bernard Rimland, Ph.D.

My own autistic son, Mark, was born in 1956, a screaming, implacable, cuddle-resistant infant who would not tolerate being picked up, or put down. I was then three years beyond my Ph.D. in psychology and had never seen or heard the word "autism." Neither had our pediatrician, who had been in practice for 35 years. It wasn't until Mark was two that my wife remembered reading in one of her old college textbooks about a youngster who looked through people rather than at them, repeated radio commercials and nursery rhymes without engaging in communicative speech, and spent hours in rocking and other pointless rituals. We found that old textbook, and there I saw the word *autism* for the first time.

It is estimated that in those days autism occurred once or twice in every 10,000 live births. But the prevalence was slowly rising. In the late 1980s I summarized the research on the prevalence of autism in an article I wrote for the *Autism Research Review,* and reported the average from a number of then-recent studies showing that autism occurred in approximately 4.5 births out of every 10,000.

How things have changed! The most recent estimates, as seen in prevalence studies of several populations in both the U.S. and U.K., range from 45 to 68 autistic children per 10,000 live births, an increase of 1,000 to 1,500 percent in two decades! (The reasons for the increase are discussed in this book.)

Whereas 20 years ago you could rarely find anyone who had ever heard of autism, today you can hardly find anyone who does not have firsthand contact with an autistic child, perhaps in his or her own family. Things have also changed very dramatically with regard to the treatment of autism.

When our Mark was an infant, the textbooks universally held that autism was an emotional, not a physiological or biomedical disorder, and the only treatment recommendations were to give psychoanalysis or other forms of psychological therapy to the mother *and* child. The mother was required to acknowledge her guilt and to search her soul to try to discover why she hated the child and wished it had never been born. The child, in so-called "play therapy," was provided with a paper or clay image of a woman (his mother) and was encouraged to tear it to pieces, thus cathartically expressing his hostility toward the mother who was presumptively guilty of having caused his autism. A few drugs were also used with autistic children, but the idea then, as now, was not to treat autism, but to slow the child down so he could become more manageable.

Just as the prevalence of autism has increased astronomically since then, so has the number of available treatment options. The traditional medical establishment has been compelled (for the most part) to abandon its barbaric insistence that the mothers admit their guilt and engage in futile "psychotherapeutic" counseling, since it is now recognized (albeit reluctantly) that autism is caused by biomedical rather than psychological factors. Conventional medicine still, however, relies largely on drugs to treat the children, and a recent compilation by the Autism Research Institute, which I founded in 1967, shows that at least 50 drugs have been tried on the 21,350 children for whom these data were available in our files.

While we parents whose children were born in the mid-twentieth century were confronted with a true paucity of possible treatment options, the parents of children born in the late twentieth century and early twenty-first century are confronted with an overabundance of choices. How do you decide which forms of intervention you should try on your autistic child? The fact that you are looking at this book is a very good sign! You have already decided that drugging the child, giving him or her Ritalin, Mellaril, Clonidine, or any of the other harmful psychoactive drugs, is not necessarily the best course of action. You are considering options, which include natural medicine.

Stephanie Marohn has done an excellent job of assembling for you a buffet of nondrug therapeutic options that you may wish to employ in your effort to bring your child out of autism. This book provides you with detailed discussions of about a dozen approaches to the treatment of autism. The description and discussion of each treatment is based on the expertise of carefully selected and respected advocates of that approach.

The next step is not easy—deciding which of the treatment approaches are best, and most appropriate, for your child. That is a decision only you, and your family, can make. As you will see, these treatment approaches vary enormously from one another in almost every respect. I say "almost" because they all agree that drugging a child who already has many problems is not a good idea.

Study these chapters. Consider the evidence supporting each of these therapies, as presented in each chapter. Consider the logic behind each therapy, and consider your child's history and symptomatology. Before long, it will become clear to you which of these natural therapies is most appropriate for your child. And if the first approach does not work out to your satisfaction, there are others you can try that are also promising.

Stephanie Marohn has done a landmark service to the parents of autistic children by providing us with this excellent compilation of natural, nondrug treatment possibilities.

Well done!

—Bernard Rimland, Ph.D.
Director, Autism Research Institute;
Founder, Autism Society of America

Acknowledgments

My profound thanks to the health-care practitioners and researchers who provided information on their work for the natural medicine treatment chapters in the book. I am very grateful for all the time and energy you generously gave in imparting this information to me and making sure that what I wrote did justice to your work. Specifically, I thank:

Richard E. Hiltner, M.D., D.Ht.
Dietrich Klinghardt, M.D., Ph.D.
Carola M. Lage-Roy, Heilpraktikerin Homoeopathie
Lawrence Lavine, D.O., M.P.H., D.T.M.&H.
Paul Madaule, L.Ps.
Devi S. Nambudripad, M.D., D.C., L.Ac., Ph.D.
Maile Pouls, Ph.D.
Judyth Reichenberg-Ullman, N.D., M.S.W.
Zannah Steiner, C.M.P., R.M.T.
William J. Walsh, Ph.D.

Additional thanks to Maile Pouls for all the research material you passed on to me.

I am also most grateful to Bernard Rimland, Ph.D., for writing the foreword to this book and for giving us the Autism Research Institute, which provided information on alternative treatments when nobody else was providing it. ARI continues to serve as a beacon of hope for parents of children diagnosed with autism.

My appreciation to Sue Trowbridge and Dorothy Anderson for

all your hard work transcribing many interviews, and to Adrienne Fodor of the Institute for Health and Healing Resource Center in San Francisco for your research assistance.

Thanks, yet again, to my editor and friend Richard Leviton for your unwavering support.

Introduction

Autism is now an epidemic in the United States. In some places, the current incidence is 1 in 150 people, and many regions report a 1,000 percent increase in the last 15 years. These facts mean that autism is more than a genetic disorder, because the incidence of genetic disorders remains stable over time. *The Natural Medicine Guide to Autism* explores the reasons for the increase in autism and details natural medicine therapies that address the underlying causes that have produced the epidemic.

This book is here to tell parents of autistic children that you don't have to accept that there is nothing you can do for your children beyond remedial intervention to help them live more easily with their limitations. You also don't have to accept that pharmaceutical drugs are your only "treatment" option. Unlike the grim prognosis conventional medicine gives the disorder, natural medicine offers a positive, practical approach to autism: identify the imbalances in the child's system, apply therapies to correct those imbalances, and autism can be ameliorated or reversed in many cases.

The approach is based on treating the causes of an individual's condition, rather than seeking to suppress the symptoms as most drugs do. The operative word here is *individual.* Treatment tailored to the individual is the key to a successful outcome because no two people are exactly the same and no two people, even with the same diagnosis, have the exact same imbalances causing their problems. Yes, as you will learn in this book, many children with autism have basic contributing factors in common, but the imbalances these factors have created in their bodies are never precisely the same. As a result, it is necessary to identify what is happening in each individual child.

To me, this approach is common sense, and I don't understand why it isn't applied throughout the medical field. Find the imbalances. Address them. To proceed with treatment in this model, you don't have to get caught up in the debate over what causes autism. The specifics of a particular child's condition guide the way to the appropriate treatment plan.

This book is here to tell parents of autistic children that you don't have to accept that there is nothing you can do for your children beyond remedial intervention to help them live more easily with their limitations. You also don't have to accept that pharmaceutical drugs are your only "treatment" option.

Using drugs to suppress symptoms makes no sense to me because it does nothing for the condition producing the symptoms. It's like sweeping dirt under a carpet—the dirt's still there even though you don't see it. And when you keep sweeping dirt under the carpet (ongoing medication), eventually the dirt can no longer be contained and you have an exponentially bigger cleanup job than you would have had in taking the dirt out of your house with each sweeping.

The analogy of dirt is an apt one in the case of human disease because the environmental toxins to which we are all exposed have turned our bodies into chemical storehouses. Today's increasing incidence of chronic and degenerative disease is a symptom of this toxicity. Autism is no exception. The developing nervous system of an infant is even more vulnerable to toxins than the adult system is. Fortunately, natural medicine therapies have methods for detoxifying the body, as you will learn in this book.

I use the term natural medicine because these therapies work with the body, not against it. This medical model recognizes the wisdom of the body. The body has its reasons for producing the symptoms it does, and it is the job of a health-care professional to discover those reasons. On a general level, neurological symptoms could be considered a cry for help from the nervous system. The cry is calling for investigation of what is creating the distress, so it can be removed. On a more specific level, a symptom such as a persistent rash can be the body's attempt to rid itself of toxins that the liver can no longer keep up with processing. Viewed in this light, autistic symptoms that may seem irrational begin to make sense.

Another important aspect of natural medicine is the core principle upon which it operates, and that is, "Do no harm." Unlike prescription drugs, which often have side effects ranging from mild to life-threatening, the therapies detailed in this book both treat your child's condition and do so without causing your child other problems.

Natural medicine restores balance to the body at a profound level, rather than employing surface palliative measures. For this reason, I prefer the term "natural medicine" over "alternative medicine." This medical model is not "other"—it is a primary form of medicine. In the book, I sometimes use the term "holistic medicine" to avoid monotony of language. I find that term equally acceptable in that it signals the natural medicine approach of treating the whole person, rather than the parts.

Part I of the book covers the basics of autism: what it is, what causes it, and the role of vaccines and mercury in its development. The natural medicine view of autism is that it is a multicausal disorder, with a variety of contributing factors and environmental triggers in those who are susceptible. Later in the book, chapter 6 details the new discovery by researcher William J. Walsh, Ph.D., who may have identified the genetic component in autism.

Part II of the book covers a range of natural medicine treatments for autism. These are advanced therapies that demonstrate the comprehensive healing potential in the field. Based on research and interviews with physicians and other health-care practitioners, the therapeutic techniques are explained in detail and illustrated with case studies. (Contact information for the practitioners appears in appendix B: Resources.) The names of patients and the family members of patients in the case studies have been changed, except in those instances in which both a first and last name appear. In these cases, the person involved gave permission to use his or her real name.

Although the focus of this book is on autism in children, the treatments discussed can be beneficial for adults with autism, too. I sincerely hope that this book is of service to you in your quest to find the help you need.

Natural Medicine Therapies

The accompanying table lists the therapies covered in each of the chapters in Part II. The main therapies of the chapters are reflected in the chapter titles. As natural medicine is a multimodal approach, however, the practitioners featured use multiple therapies, so the majority of the chapters cover a number of different treatment modalities.

Chapter	Health Practitioner	Therapies/Testing
4	Maile Pouls, Ph.D.	24-hour urinalysis Hair analysis Enzyme therapy Nutritional supplements Digestive/intestinal therapy Heavy metal detoxification/oral chelation
5	Devi S. Nambudripad, M.D., D.C., L.Ac., Ph.D.	NAET (allergy testing and elimination; includes MRT, muscle response testing)
6	William J. Walsh, Ph.D.	Urine and blood testing Biochemical therapy Metallothionein dysfunction therapy Digestive/intestinal therapy Gluten-free/casein-free diet Heavy metal detoxification
7	Judyth Reichenberg-Ullman, N.D., M.S.W. Richard E. Hiltner, M.D., D.Ht.	Constitutional homeopathy Homeopathic nosodes

Covered in Part II

	Carola M. Lage-Roy, Naturopath-Homeopath	(Isopathy) for vaccine Clearing and as vaccine alternatives
	Philip Incao, M.D.	Homeopathy to treat childhood illnesses
8	Lawrence Lavine, D.O., M.P.H., D.T.M.&H.	Cranial osteopathy Homeopathy Isopathy NAET
9	Zannah Steiner, C.M.P., R.M.T.	CranioSacral therapy Visceral Manipulation SomatoEmotional Release
10	Paul Madaule, L.Ps.	Tomatis method (listening training/sensory integration technique)
11	Dietrich Klinghardt, M.D., Ph.D.	Neural therapy ART (autonomic response testing) Chelation/heavy metal detoxification Homeopathic nosodes for vaccine clearing Gluten-free/casein-free diet Family systems therapy

Part I

The Basics of Autism

1 What Is Autism?

"You know, Mommy, the world is full of sounds. When I listen to them, I realize that the sounds make patterns, and the patterns all turn into music in my head. Sometimes when you call me, I don't hear you because I'm listening to the music."[1]

—Miles, 5 years old, recovered from the autism diagnosed at 19 months

After long being regarded as a mental illness or emotional maladjustment, autism is now recognized as a biological disorder, meaning that it is due to organic rather than psychological causes. More specifically, autism is a neurological or brain-based developmental disorder that particularly manifests in problems in cognition, communication, and interaction. The onset typically occurs before three years of age.

Despite the consensus of biological causality, the American Psychiatric Association's criteria remain the standard for an autism diagnosis, and autism is still classified as a mental disorder in the *Diagnostic and Statistical Manual of Mental Disorders-Fourth Edition (DSM-IV)*, the diagnostic bible for psychiatric disorders. As the criteria paint a portrait of the disorder, I include a summary here.

For a diagnosis of autism, according to the *DSM-IV* criteria, a person must have at least six items from the three areas delineated below, with at least two from the first area and one each from the other two.[2]

1. Impairment in social interaction
   - impairment in nonverbal behaviors related to social interaction, such as eye contact and facial expression
   - failure to develop peer relationships
   - lack of spontaneous sharing of enjoyment or interests, as evidenced by showing or pointing out objects
   - lack of social or emotional reciprocity

2. Impairment in communication
   - delayed or nonexistent language development
   - impairment in conversation abilities if language is present
   - stereotypic, repetitive language or idiosyncratic language
   - lack of make-believe or social imitative play

3. Repetitive and stereotyped behavior, interests, and activities
   - abnormally intense preoccupation with one or more interests
   - seemingly inflexible adherence to routines or rituals
   - stereotyped and repetitive mannerisms, such as hand or finger flapping or twisting, or whole-body movements
   - preoccupation with object parts

While the *DSM-IV* description is a good starting place for understanding what autism looks like, there are many symptoms and conditions associated with the disorder that are not reflected in these criteria. This is especially true when autism is considered from a biological rather than a behavioral perspective, which involves looking beyond the outward signs to what is happening on the inside.

For example, many children with autism suffer from allergies, nutritional deficiencies, and/or intestinal overgrowth of the yeast-like fungus *Candida*. Many also have weakened immunity or autoimmune problems. See the sidebar (pages 6-7) for an expanded list of the symptoms, behaviors, and conditions that have been found to be associated with autism.

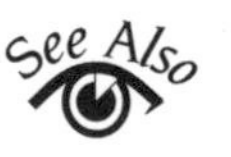

For more about the symptoms of autism and their correlation with other factors involved in the disorder, see sidebars in chapters 5 and 6.

An aspect of autism that has fascinated many is what is known as "islets of ability." Autism pioneer Leo Kanner (see "The History of Autism," which follows) coined the term to refer to the advanced skill areas of autistic children. The most well documented "islets" are in drawing, music, calendar calculation, and rote memory. Unusual drawing ability, perfect pitch, the ability to play an instrument that one has never been taught, and the ability to play a complex piece after hearing it only once are all examples of islets of ability.[3]

Another positive aspect of autism may arise from behavior that often drives family members to distraction. Temple Grandin, who was autistic from an early age and provides rare insight into the experience of autism in her book *Emergence: Labeled Autistic,* points out a potential benefit of the intense preoccupation with certain objects that is characteristic of autism. "High functioning autistic adults, who are able to live independently and keep a job, often have work that is in the same field of interest as their childhood fixations."[4] In her case, an early obsession with livestock equipment turned into a creative adult profession as a designer of such equipment.

Grandin also illuminates the function of the puzzling, repetitive, almost ritualistic behaviors in which many autistic children engage. "I, as an autistic person, reacted in a fixated behavior pattern in order to reduce arousal to my overly stimulated nervous system. . . . By concentrating on the fixation, [autistic-type children] block out other stimulation which they cannot handle."[5] Of her sensitivity to sound, Grandin says, "Sometimes I heard and understood, and other times sounds or speech reached my brain like the unbearable noise of an onrushing freight train."[6]

Donna Williams provides another glimpse into the inaccessible world of autism. She, like Temple Grandin, was autistic from early childhood and went on to write a book about the experience, entitled *Nobody Nowhere: The Extraordinary Autobiography of an Autistic.* She, too, offers an explanation for the fixed behavior patterns and repetitive actions. "The constant change of most things never seemed to give me any chance to prepare myself for

Symptoms, Behaviors, and Conditions Associated with Autism

- anxiety
- attention deficit
- distractibility
- hyperactivity
- hypersensitivity to:
  - sound
  - light
  - touch
  - certain foods
  - environmental toxins
  - vaccines
- hypersensitivity or imperviousness to pain
- seeming lack of awareness of danger
- impulsivity
- self-stimulatory behavior (stimming) such as rocking or twirling
- hand flapping and other repetitive movements
- rhythmic rocking
- walking on tiptoe
- severe language deficits
- loud, monotone voice
- lack of use of the pronoun 'I,' referring to self in the third person
- echolalia (repeating others' words or phrases)
- prosody (singsong speech)
- abnormal nystagmus (eye movement)
- islets of ability (perfect pitch, unusual drawing or musical talent, calculation or rote memory skills, etc.)
- preoccupation with light switches or other objects
- spinning objects repetitively
- unusual and intense interests
- repetitive acts and thoughts (stereotypies, mannerisms, perseverations, obsessions, and compulsions)
- using someone's hand or arm as a tool, as if it is not attached to a human being
- absence of pointing
- lack of shared attention (showing or pointing to something)
- no playing peek-a-boo
- impaired nonverbal behaviors (eye contact, etc.)
- incomprehension of gesture
- impaired social interaction
- impaired communication
- seeming lack of interest in people
- seeming unresponsiveness to verbal cues (parents may suspect deafness, but hearing tests normal)
- blank remoteness

- seemingly expressionless face
- resistance to change
- tantrums or odd behavior in reaction to sudden change or for no apparent reason
- laughing, crying, or showing other emotion for no apparent reason
- lack of spontaneity
- lack of curiosity
- poor appetite
- allergies
- inability to process casein and gluten
- fungal overgrowth
- digestive problems
- leaky gut syndrome
- nutritional deficiencies
- autoimmune problems
- weakened immunity
- chronic or frequent colds, flu, and ear and other infections
- heavy metal toxicity

In addition to these indicators, research has discovered abnormalities in the brains of people with autism, variously in the cerebellum, limbic system, frontal cortex, and amygdala, and in brain waves. Studies have also found elevated blood levels of the neurotransmitter serotonin in autistic people, but reduced uptake in the brain may mean that the availability of this vital nerve messenger is actually limited.[7]

them. Because of this I found pleasure and comfort in doing the same things over and over again."[8]

Jerry, who was five years old when Leo Kanner diagnosed his autism, painted a painful picture of what it was like for him as a child. At the age of 31, he told psychiatrist J. R. Bemporad about his experience of autism, which Dr. Bemporad reported as follows:

"According to Jerry, his childhood experience could be summarized as consisting of two predominant experiential states: confusion and terror. The recurrent theme that ran though all of Jerry's recollections was that of living in a frightening world presenting painful stimuli that could not be mastered. Noises were unbearably loud, smells overpowering. Nothing seemed constant; everything was unpredictable and strange."[9]

In Their Own Words

"Sara has an exceptional memory, particularly for dates and what happened on those dates. . . . She was a big [Eduard] Munch fan for a long time and I found an old Munch calendar in a remainder bin in a bookstore. . . . She spent an entire weekend filling in the events of every day of that preceding year—things that we had forgotten entirely. And when we checked back in my datebook or with friends, she was absolutely dead on as to what had happened, where we'd been, and even what people had worn."[10]

—Sara's mother

"I remember when [Sara] was four, maybe five years old, being inside the house, in the winter, with music on the stereo that was quite loud, and conversations going on, and trying to talk to her, and she reacted really strongly, wanted us to be quiet so she could hear the airplane. Of course, we couldn't hear the airplane. Everyone was quiet. We turned the stereo off, opened the door, and listened really carefully, and we could hear a small plane somewhere in the distance. But she heard that through everything."[11]

—Sara's father

"My bed was also surrounded and totally encased by tiny spots that I called stars. . . . I have since learned that they are actually air particles, yet my vision was so hypersensitive that they often became a hypnotic foreground with the rest of 'the world' fading away. . . . The hypnotic fascination I had for the spots in the air left me with very little sensation of my own body except for the shock and repulsion of the invasion of physical closeness. . . . I learned to tolerate being hugged . . . being hugged hurt me and . . . It felt like I was being burned."[12]

—Donna Williams, university-educated author of *Nobody Nowhere: The Extraordinary Autobiography of an Autistic,* among other books

Who Gets Autism?

Today, over 500,000 people in the United States have autism. That number is increasing daily at an alarming rate, prompting many professionals to declare that we are in the midst of an epidemic of autism.[13] The current incidence rate for the disorder varies, depending on the source consulted. The Centers for Disease Control and Prevention (CDC) places the number at 1 in 500 in the general population, and 1 in 150 in some places in the country (notably Brick Township, New Jersey, home to a toxic landfill).[14] The U.S. Department of Health and Human Services, as represented in the Surgeon General's report on mental health, places the number at 1 to 2 in 1,000.[15]

The American Academy of Child and Adolescent Psychiatry cites "a conservative estimate for the prevalence of autism" of 1 per 2,000 people, and 1 per 1,000 if Asperger's syndrome is included.[16] The incidence rate, according to the Autism Research Institute, is now 1 in 160 to 200, up from 1 in 2,500 in the 1980s.[17] The American Medical Association (AMA) states that as many as one in five children today have a neurodevelopmental condition such as autism, a learning disorder, or attention deficit/hyperactivity disorder.[18]

While the exact numbers may differ, no one argues that there has been an enormous increase in the incidence of autism. Autism now affects 1 in 150 to 500 children in the United States. The incidence has risen by as much as 1000 percent in the last 15 to 20 years.[19] One of the places where the 1000-percent increase has been documented is California. That percentage may be more than other places simply because the state keeps excellent records. It has what may be the world's best database on autism and other developmental disorders.[20]

The cause for the increase is the subject of great debate and controversy. Some say it is an issue of awareness, but many long-time teachers, who have seen the sharp increase of autistic behaviors in their classrooms, independent of diagnosis, would contest this view. Many people—both autism experts and parents of autistic children—blame the increase on the rise in the number and nature of vaccines given to children. This topic is explored at length in chapter 3, but suffice it to say here that the number of vaccines that children receive in the first two years of life has gone up from 8 in 1980 to 22 in the year 2001.[21] In addition, the rise in autism has occurred in all countries that follow the World Health Organization's vaccination guidelines.[22]

Other autism statistics of interest are:[23]

- Four out of five people with autism are male.

- One in ten of those with autism show unusual abilities in art, music, calculation, or memory.

- The risk of developing autism is 25 times greater for those with an autistic sibling than for those without an autistic sibling.

- The risk of developing autism is 375 times greater for those who have an identical twin with autism.

- One doctor's clinical analysis revealed that in 60 percent of his autistic patients, their birth involved the use of the Pitocin (a drug to speed the contractions during labor); only 20 percent of all births involve Pitocin.

Types of Autism

In addition to the diagnosis of autism, other diagnostic labels are currently applied to children with autistic symptoms and characteristics. There are many labels used; following are a few of the more common. A holistic approach does not use such diagnoses to determine the appropriate treatment course, focusing instead on the particular manifestations and underlying imbalances in the individual patient. Further, the diagnoses are not distinct and, in many cases, one could be used as well as another. Many autistic children receive these labels, however, so it's helpful to know to what they refer.

Pervasive developmental disorder (PDD): This is a general term for autism and other developmental disorders that involve severe impairment in the three areas cited as diagnostic criteria for autism; that is, impairment in social interaction, communication impairment, and repetitive or stereotyped behaviors, interests, or activities.

Autistic spectrum disorder (ASD): This term encompasses the varieties of autism and reflects the relatively new view of the disorder; that is, that it manifests in varying degrees of severity along a continuum from mild to severe and in varying forms depending on which neurological functions are most affected.

Many people—both autism experts and parents of autistic children—blame the increase in autism on the rise in the number and nature of vaccines given to children. The number of vaccines that children receive in the first two years of life has gone up from 8 in 1980 to 22 in the year 2001.

Asperger's syndrome: In what is considered a milder form of autism than classic autism, language development is not as affected and the child may even be precociously verbal.

Atypical autism: This refers to a departure from the manifestations of classic autism in the three areas of impairment: impairment in social interaction, impairment in communication, and repetitive and stereotyped behavior, interests, and activities. Children with atypical autism exhibit effects in only two of the three areas.

Names are also used to distinguish the nature of onset. A diagnosis of classic autism, known as Kanner's autism, early infantile autism, childhood autism, or autistic disorder, generally involves the onset of abnormalities within the first two years of the child's life. Some practitioners make the distinction between classic autism and what they term regressive autism, meaning there was a period of normal development before the onset of abnormalities.

Many parents report that their child was fine until around 15 to 18 months. Most children are not diagnosed until they are at least three, however, because developmental delays are more obvious by that time. Diagnosis in autism is confusing, and made more confusing by the fact that the spectrum or continuum type of labels are in the process of being defined.

In Their Own Words

"My story, which is a really common one and a really sad one, is that I couldn't get anyone to accept that there was something wrong. I would always hear the same old line: 'Every child develops differently. You're worrying too much. You're overprotective.' I think parents know when their child isn't connecting with them. [Sara] would pull away when I would try to cuddle her. I didn't have a whole lot of experience—she's my only child—but I knew it wasn't right."[24]

—mother of Sara, who was finally diagnosed with autism at the age of 12

Autism Myths

The following are common myths about autism.[25] The fact that myths related to the obsolete view of autism as a mental illness persist reveals how well disseminated that view was. Only equally good dissemination of the biological reality of autism will at last dispel that stigmatizing notion. The persistence of all of these myths indicates the need for education of the general public about this disorder.

Myth: Bad parenting causes autism.

This formerly widely held view has been thoroughly debunked in the scientific community. It is now known that autism is a neurological and developmental disorder, not one caused by psychological factors. "Poor mother/child bonding, if it is to be associated with Autism at all, must be seen as effect rather than a cause of Autism," states Uta Frith, author of *Autism: Explaining the Enigma.*[26]

Myth: Children with autism choose to live in their own world.

Choice has nothing to do with it. Neurological dysfunction is the source of autistic children's manner of interacting with the world. Autistic behaviors arise from the different "wiring" inherent to the disorder. Hypersensitivity to sound, light, touch, and environmental factors as a result of neurological problems are additional features that often make such interaction stressful and even painful.

Myth: Children with autism avoid eye contact.

This is not necessarily the case. Many do make eye contact, although it may be done in a different manner from children who are not autistic. Uta Frith explains that they are not avoiding the gaze, as is typically believed, but rather lack understanding of and the ability to use the "language of the eyes," a vital component of social communication. "The child neither looks away at the right time, nor meets the gaze when this would be expected. . . . Whatever causes the inability to use the language of the eyes has nothing to do with avoidance of human contact."[27] As you will learn later in this book, the problem of gaze and other attributes of autism are often improved or disappear with natural medicine therapies that resolve the biological issues involved in an individual case.

Myth: People with autism are actually geniuses, or savants like Dustin Hoffman's character in the film Rain Man.

Only 1 in 10 people with autism have what are termed "islets of ability or intelligence," such as unusual artistic or musical talent or extraordinary calculation or memory skills. Like other children, the IQs of children with autism range throughout the scale, with only a small percentage falling in the lower and upper ranges. Dysfunction in certain areas of mental processing are common to autistic children.

Myth: Children with autism don't speak.

On the contrary, many develop "good functional language," while most others learn to communicate through sign language, pictures, computers, or electronic devices.[28] As with other features of autism, the more the biological factors can be ameliorated, the greater the possibility that the child will attain normal language skills.

Myth: Children with autism could talk if they wanted to.

One of the areas greatly affected by the neurological problems and developmental delays of autism is speech. Autistic muteness and lack of verbal response to questions is not a matter of stubbornness or noncompliance, but the result of developmental impairment of speech.

Myth: Children with autism can't show affection.

The Autism Society of America calls this "one of the most devastating myths for families." As with eye contact, the differences in their "wiring" may make autistic children express their love and affection differently from other children. This does not mean they can't give and receive love. Family members need to be willing to meet the child on her terms and recognize her capacity to connect.

Myth: Children with autism lack feelings and emotions.

Clearly, this is not the case, as evidenced by temper tantrums and happy laughter. The fact that many autistic children lack affect in their facial expressions and speak in a flat tone if they do speak aids in the survival of this myth. As with the myth above, it is the communication of emotions, not their existence, that is the issue. All aspects of communication are problematic for autistic children due to their neurological dysfunction and developmental delays, and emotional communication is no exception. A seeming disregard for other people's feelings also fuels this myth. The disregard does not indicate, however, that the child lacks emotions. One of the neurological impairments of autism is a lack of imagination, thus the child cannot imagine what another person is thinking or feeling.

Myth: Children with autism are just spoiled kids with behavior problems.

This myth brings the curse of autism back to the parents' door. It reflects the tenaciousness of the psychological model. It also shows a lack of understanding of the profound and far-reaching effects of neurological impairment on behavior, mood, and motor and language development, among other areas.

Myth: Autism is forever. If the condition improves significantly, it means the child was misdiagnosed and does not have autism.

This is a myth that persists in the conventional medical and psychiatric world, with its dismal prognosis for autism. Given the lack of means to reverse or ameliorate the biological factors involved in autism, the prognosis is understandable and the myth goes unchallenged.

As this book demonstrates, however, improvement and even reversal are possible when you can address the underlying factors in treatment. Many children who strictly met the criteria for a diagnosis of autism experienced significant improvement with natural medicine approaches. On the more conservative end of treatment, methods such as behavior modification, speech therapy, and occupational therapy are well known to produce improvement in autistic children.

In Their Own Words

"[T]here are still many parents, and, yes, professionals, too, who believe that 'once autistic, always autistic.' This dictum has meant sad and sorry lives for many children diagnosed, as I was in early life, as autistic. To these people it is incomprehensible that the characteristics of autism can be modified and controlled....I am living proof that they can."[29]

—Temple Grandin, Ph.D., livestock handling equipment designer and co-author of *Emergence: Labeled Autistic*

The History of Autism

The word 'autism' derives from the Greek *auto* (self) and *-ismos* (condition). Psychiatrist Eugen Bleuler coined the term in 1911 in reference to an aspect of schizophrenia characterized by withdrawal from the outside world into the self. In the 1940s, in the first papers published on the disorder, Leo Kanner and Hans Asperger both borrowed the term to describe autism. Kanner's description of the disorder became the classic autism of today, while Asperger's description became what is now called Asperger's syndrome, despite the fact that his account was of classic autism rather than the less severe form that came to bear his name.

The psychiatric roots of the label *autism* continued in the long-standing belief that psychological factors were the cause of autism. This psychogenic theory, otherwise known as the "refrigerator mother" theory, which held that the mother's lack of emotional engagement with her child produced autism, enjoyed cachet for decades. In the 1960s, Bruno Bettelheim, a psychoanalyst and proponent of the refrigerator mother theory, went so far as to advocate removing the child from the parents as treatment. He detailed his views in his book *The Empty Fortress: Infantile Autism and the Birth of the Self*, which for some time was considered a classic work on autism.[30] The psychogenic theory of autism began to topple with the publication in 1964 of *Infantile Autism*, by Bernard Rimland, Ph.D. This book ushered in the era of biological causation.

The following years saw the emergence of evidence that indisputably disproved the psychogenic theory. Three compelling points in this large body of evidence are: autism is not associated with dysfunctional families, but strikes across families and cultures; the developmental abnormalities that result from extreme emotional rejection and social deprivation are different from autistic abnormalities, and since even severe deprivation fails to produce autism, it is hardly likely that a somewhat cool mother would do so; and one-third of adolescents with autism suffer from seizures, which indicates an organic problem, a brain abnormality.[31]

While the psychogenic theory, which brought so much unnecessary pain to parents of autistic children, is no longer considered valid, vestiges of it persist in public attitude and in professional circles. The survival of the previous myths of autism speak to the stigma of mental illness that still surrounds autism in the general public. As noted earlier, the American Psychiatric Association continues to classify autism as a mental disorder and its diagnostic criteria remain the standard.

While some medical dictionaries have modified their definitions of autism, a classic reference, *Taber's Cyclopedic Medical Dictionary*, still defines infantile autism as "a syndrome appearing in childhood with symptoms of self-absorption, inaccessibility, aloneness, inability to relate, highly repetitive play and rage reactions if interrupted, predilection for rhythmical movements, and many language disturbances," with unknown etiology.[32]

The description and the omission of even possible organic causality leave the psychological bias in place.

In the early days of psychiatric diagnosis, autistic people were often labeled schizophrenic. Whatever the label, they were considered ineducable, and institutionalization was a common fate. While the views regarding educability have changed, conventional wisdom still holds that autism is not a treatable disorder, that the best you can do is train autistic children out of some of their limitations. A *Newsweek* cover story on autism in July 2000 reflected this view, focusing on a form of behavior modification as the treatment of choice and stating that "most [autistic children] end up in institutions by the age of 13."[33]

As those involved in natural medicine approaches to autism know and as you will learn in this book, treatment holds the possibility for much more than simply working with the limitations.

2 *Causes and Contributing* Factors

The cause of autism is officially stated as unknown. Among the various theories and conjectures, the one area of agreement is that there is a genetic component that renders certain children susceptible or vulnerable. In a review of recent advances in autism research published in the *Journal of Psychiatry and Neuroscience,* the study's author concluded that "the prevailing view is that autism is caused by a pathophysiologic process arising from the interaction of an early environmental insult and a genetic predisposition."[34]

Similarly, in holistic medicine, a widely accepted view is that autism is a genetic disorder triggered by environmental factors. (*Environmental* in this usage simply means not genetic, so injuries and nutritional deficiencies from a poor diet, for example, fall in the environmental category, as do the effects of viruses and vaccines.) As with other illnesses, natural medicine practitioners regard the development of autism in those who are susceptible as multicausal rather than the consequence of a single cause. When the body is exposed to one too many stress factors, illness results.

The fact that the incidence of autism has increased to epidemic proportions is an indication that genetics cannot be the sole cause of the disorder. By definition, genetic disorders affect a stable percentage of the population. A huge jump in the number of cases signals that other factors are involved.

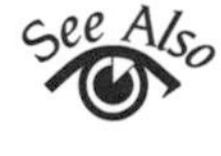

Thus far, research has failed to isolate the genetic component in autism. With a new discovery by William J. Walsh, Ph.D., however, that may no longer be true. See chapter 6 for details of this hopeful development in the quest to end autism.

As you learned in chapter 1, there are numerous symptoms and conditions associated with autism. It is difficult to determine the causal relationship among them. Was the child born with a weak immune system? Did that make him susceptible to developing allergies? Or did digestive dysfunction come first, followed by fungal overgrowth and the development of allergies? Did an inborn weakness make him particularly sensitive to the viral and heavy-metal load in vaccines? Did in utero toxic exposure result in him being born with an already high toxic load that meant even a relatively minor exposure after birth was more than his body could handle? Did he have five different factors that combined to provide the trigger for autism?

It is nearly impossible to answer these questions definitively, but, fortunately, the answers aren't necessary in order to proceed with treatment. Identifying what is happening in the child now is what matters. While treatment at this time cannot remove the genetic component in autism, treating the underlying conditions and reversing the effects of the environmental influences can improve or even eliminate autistic symptoms. The first step, then, is to identify all of the factors involved in an individual case of autism, for no two children have exactly the same set of underlying imbalances. Again, whether these imbalances together contributed to the development of the autism, arose as a result of the autism, or were caused by the other imbalances may not be clear.

The factors that may play a role in triggering or worsening autism include: cranial distortions from birth trauma; vaccine-related problems; heavy metal and chemical toxicity; immune dysfunction; allergies; nutritional deficiencies or imbalances; and digestive problems, including fungal overgrowth. Some doctors, researchers, and parents of autistic children firmly view some of these factors as causes. Whatever their role, one or all of the factors are commonly present in autistic children.

The natural medicine model recognizes the wisdom of the body and its continual movement toward healing itself. In this regard, the manifestations of autism, as inexplicable as they appear, may reflect the body's attempt to cope with these abnormal factors. For example, Zannah Steiner, C.M.P., R.M.T., notes in chapter 9 that autistic head-banging may be an attempt to ease the pressure that birth-induced cranial distortions create in the head.

The first step is to identify all of the factors involved in an individual case of autism, for no two children have exactly the same set of underlying imbalances.

Birth trauma is discussed at length in chapters 8 and 9. The role of vaccines and the heavy metal mercury is covered in chapter 3. This chapter focuses on the remaining factors linked to autism. The interrelationship of these factors adds to the complexity of the disorder. I begin with a discussion of toxins because they may be central in weakening the system and leaving it vulnerable to the development of the other factors and autism itself.

Toxins

Toxic overload may be one of the reasons for the current autism epidemic. Humans today are exposed to an unprecedented number of chemicals. Testing of anyone on Earth, no matter how remote the area in which they live, will reveal that they are carrying at least 250 chemical contaminants in their body fat.[35]

The onslaught of chemicals begins in the womb, with the transmission of toxins from the toxic mother to the fetus, and continues with breast-feeding. An infant in the United States or Europe imbibes "the maximum recommended lifetime dose of dioxin" in only six months of nursing. Dioxin, a pesticide by-product, is one of the most toxic substances on Earth.[36] Nursing Inuit mothers in the Arctic have some of the highest PCB levels in breast milk in the world due to the large quantity of marine mammal fat in their diet.[37]

Two recent reports, one by the Greater Boston Physicians for Social Responsibility and the other published in *U.S. News and World Report*, independently arrived at the same conclusion, "that chemicals in our environment may play a profound role in the increased incidence of birth and developmental defects, particularly the increase in attentional problems, autism, and learning disabilities."[38] Evidence is mounting that chemical compounds called neurotoxicants are at least in part responsible for the fact that one in six children in the United States now suffers from autism, aggression, dyslexia, or attention deficit hyperactivity disorder (ADHD), according to the Learning Disabilities Association of America.[39]

Contributing Factors in Autism

The following may play a role in triggering or worsening autism:

- cranial distortions from birth trauma
- vaccines
- heavy metal and chemical toxicity
- viruses or viral overload
- immune dysfunction
- digestive problems, including fungal overgrowth
- food allergies, particularly to gluten and casein
- sensitivity to food additives
- nutritional deficiencies/imbalances

In their report, *In Harm's Way—Toxic Threats to Child Development*, the Greater Boston Physicians for Social Responsibility summarize research about in utero and childhood exposure to developmental neurotoxicants, which they define as "chemicals that are toxic to the developing brain." These include lead, mercury, cadmium, manganese, nicotine, pesticides (many of which are commonly used in homes and schools), dioxin and PCBs (polychlorinated biphenyls; both PCBs and dioxin stay in the food chain once they enter it, as they pervasively have), and solvents used in paint, glue, and cleaning products.

The report notes that in one year alone (1997), industrial plants released more than a billion pounds of these chemicals directly into the environment (air, water, and land). Further, almost 75 percent of the top 20 chemicals (those released in the largest quantities) are known or suspected to be neurotoxicants.[40] Other sources report that of 70,000 different chemicals being used commercially only 10 percent have been tested for their effect on the nervous system.[41]

Among the findings in the *In Harm's Way* report are:[42]

- Fetal exposure to large amounts of methylmercury results in mental retardation and gait and visual disturbances. A smaller fetal exposure, as from the pregnant mother regularly eating fish, has been linked to apparently permanent impairments in language, attention, and memory.

- Women who smoke during pregnancy bear children who are at risk for learning disorders and attention and IQ deficits. Even secondary smoke exposure during pregnancy puts the child at risk for impairment in language skills, speech, and intelligence.

- Fetal exposure to PCBs has adverse effects on brain development and results in later hyperactivity and IQ and attention deficits.

- Chlorpyrifos (Dursban), a widely used pesticide of the organophosphate class, decreases the synthesis of DNA in the developing brain, which results in fewer brain cells than normal.

- Solvent exposure during development has been linked to hyperactivity, structural birth defects, lower IQs, and learning, memory, and attention deficits.

In a study of 26 autistic children, Stephen B. Edelson, M.D., director of the Edelson Center for Environmental and Preventive Medicine in Atlanta, Georgia, found that 90 percent of them "showed evidence of toxic chemical exposure," and 90 percent of their mothers had been exposed during pregnancy to higher than usual amounts of toxic household and industrial chemicals. The chemicals included formaldehyde, pesticides, and toxins from paint, ceramics, ant and flea sprays, and new carpets. Dr. Edelson also found that all of the children had allergies, neurotransmitter (brain messenger) imbalances, nutritional deficiencies, and immune system abnormalities; 40 percent of them had nutrient absorption problems.[43]

It is clear that from conception onward children are exposed to toxins. Even the new carpet in your home can poison your baby in utero or after he's born. Outgassing from new carpets is a well-known phenomenon; the glue used and the foam carpet pads are particularly toxic. "The multiple studies which have proposed or which have found new carpets in the prenatal period to be a significant risk factor [for autism] suggest an additional component supporting adverse environmental issues," states Lawrence Lavine, D.O., whose work with autism is covered in chapter 8.[44]

While there is ample evidence that the toxic load we are all carrying is having serious effects on even the health of otherwise healthy people, the autistic child may be further compromised by the additional load of other factors that place stress on the body. These include any of the other factors discussed in this chapter and the next. For instance, when a susceptible child's body, already loaded with toxins from fetal exposure, is subjected to a vaccine containing not only multiple viruses but also a mercury-based preservative, that may be sufficient to tip the balance into autism. The neurotoxins and the viral load is too much for the beleaguered body to handle, and the nervous and immune systems break down.

Inefficient liver detoxification, a feature in many cases of autism, may contribute to the autistic child's inability to handle the toxic load. The liver is the body's main detoxification organ and processes toxins for elimination from the body. When the liver does not properly process toxins, whether due to genetic weakness in the liver detoxification system or toxic overload that the liver cannot keep up with, toxic buildup occurs.

The evidence suggests that the increase in autism is due to the environmental onslaught (including the increasing number of vaccines children receive) to which we are all now subject and which has been steadily increasing over the past 50 years. Some people argue that what we are seeing is not "true" autism. It may be, however, that Kanner's classic autism was not as prevalent in his day because the genetic susceptibility was not triggered as often by environmental factors. Now, the triggers are many, and so autism has reached epidemic proportions. The environmental component was probably not factored in to the equation in the mid-1900s, when the disorder was brought to more widespread awareness, because environmental toxicity was not as big a problem or as recognized as it is today.

Has autism always had the environmental trigger component? We don't know the answer to that, but it certainly appears that what we have going on now involves such triggers. Our bodies have not evolved to the point of being able to handle the level of toxins to which we are exposed—witness the growing incidence of degenerative disease, including cancer, which is clearly a disease of toxicity.

It is hard enough for the adult body, but infants' developing systems are particularly vulnerable. While we can't at present fully protect them from exposure to the toxins in our air, water, and earth, it is heartbreaking that we don't protect them in the areas in which we do have control. Instead, we purposely inject their little bodies with a known neurotoxin (mercury) and multiple vaccines. This is unnecessary for a number of reasons, and there are safe alternatives to the current vaccination policy (see chapter 7).

Perhaps in the future, our bodies will have developed a greater ability to process toxins and withstand the onslaught, and the rates of autism, cancer, and other diseases will go down. But do we really want to adapt to this toxic situation? Wouldn't it be better to clean up our dirty nest?

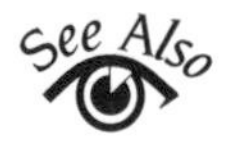

For an in-depth discussion of mercury toxicity, see chapter 3.

Immune Dysfunction

One of the most consistent findings in research on autism is the presence of immunological abnormalities.[45] This fact is made more significant by the increasing understanding in scientific circles of the interrelationship between the nervous and immune systems.[46] "[E]arly and severe derailments of the immune system can lead to profound neurological damage. Such derailments have been known to occur in conjunction with severe environmental insults, such as pre- or post-natal viral infections, or through vaccinations," states Laura J. Ruede, of the Autism Autoimmunity Project in Lake Hiawatha, New Jersey.

A genetic weakness in the immune system may make it more vulnerable to environmental insults and thus more susceptible to malfunction. Ruede notes that "A viral 'insult' in predisposed persons can ultimately lead to a state of autoimmunity, or continuous immune reaction against the body's own tissues. Antibodies against brain and other body elements have been detected in autism. . . ."[47]

The Autism Autoimmunity Project is dedicated to raising money for research into what they term "immune-based autism." Whether immune breakdown is a corollary or a cause of autism, it is undeniable that immune dysfunction is frequently present. It is important to note that the toxic onslaught previously discussed may be one of the environmental insults that contribute to immune breakdown, as may vaccines and viruses. Research scientist Uta Frith states: "The theory that psychotic illness can be due to immune dysfunction and/or viral infection has particular justification in the area of Autism. It has been shown . . . that a virus infection in a young child preceded the onset of typical symptoms of Autism, before which there was a period of apparently normal development. . . . If the central nervous system becomes infected at a critical time, either before or after birth, Autism may result."[48]

Digestive Problems

British gastroenterologist Andrew J. Wakefield sparked a huge controversy with a research article in the February 1998 issue of the prestigious medical journal the *Lancet,* in which he suggested there may be a connection between pervasive developmental disorder and gastrointestinal problems possibly brought on by the MMR (measles, mumps, and rubella) vaccine.[49] Dr. Wakefield became the target of virulent criticism and attack. With subsequent research, he and his colleagues had, as of April 2001, tested nearly 200 children and found the same pattern in the great majority of them. He reported their findings before the U.S. Congressional Oversight Committee on Government Reform, which was investigating the autism and vaccine connection. Here is a portion of his testimony to the committee:

> "In summary, primary intestinal pathology may be a significant part of the disease process in a large, but as yet undefined, proportion of the children with autism. In the great majority of autistic children who have been investigated appropriately, according to their intestinal symptoms, there is inflammatory pathology, the features of which are consistent with an autoimmune mucosal lesion in both the large and small intestine. We propose that this intestinal disease makes a major contribution to the developmental/behavioral pathology in affected children."[50]

These findings were consistent with a viral cause for this syndrome, noted Dr. Wakefield. In addition, in 93 percent of the autistic children studied, both measles virus genes and protein were present in intestinal tissues, as well as in swollen ileal lymph nodes, which was one of the features of the intestinal pathology pattern he identified.

Dr. Wakefield is careful to say that it has not been proven that the measles virus present in the intestines of these children is from MMR vaccines. He is in the process of conducting research to determine that. Given that many of the parents of the children in the study report that their child's behavioral symptoms began *after* MMR vaccination and the fact that the vast majority had not had measles infection, it seems likely that the vaccines are the source of the virus in the intestinal tissue.

Another common digestive problem found in autistic children may also contribute to the neurological symptoms of autism. In an article entitled "Candida-Caused Autism?" Dr. Bernard Rimland, director of the Autism Research Institute in San Diego, California, summarized the available information on the role of an overgrowth of the yeast-like fungus *Candida* in the intestines.[51] (The term *candidiasis* is typically used to refer to a systemic overgrowth of *Candida*; an overgrowth in the mouth is called oral thrush.) A *Candida* overgrowth indicates intestinal dysbiosis, an imbalance of the flora that normally inhabit the intestines.

Repeated use of antibiotics is one of the factors that can cause a fungal overgrowth, as they kill both harmful bacteria and the beneficial bacteria that keep *Candida* in check. As many autistic children have compromised immunity, they get frequent illnesses, from colds and flu to recurrent or chronic ear infections. Many have been on numerous courses of antibiotics by the time they are two years old. In these children, fungal overgrowth is likely. The frequent use of antifungal medications in the treatment of autism highlights the prevalence of this problem.

Although there is not enough research on the subject to draw a definite conclusion, says* Dr. Rimland, *"based on the weight of the information gathered to date, it seems to me highly probable that a small, but significant, proportion of children diagnosed as autistic are in fact victims of a severe* Candida *infection."

Although there is not enough research on the subject to draw a definite conclusion, says Dr. Rimland, "based on the weight of the information gathered to date, it seems to me highly probable that a small, but significant, proportion of children diagnosed as autistic are in fact victims of a severe *Candida* infection. I further believe that if the *Candida* infection were successfully treated in these few cases. . . . the symptoms of autism would show dramatic improvement."

Dr. Rimland estimates that 5 to 10 percent of autistic children might benefit from proper treatment for their *Candida* overgrowth.[52] Eliminating foods that "feed" *Candida* is a common treatment approach. The so-called candida diet emphasizes avoiding all forms and sources of sugar, including fruit and fruit juice, carbohydrates, and fermented yeast products.

A number of natural medicine practitioners, notably Dr. Thomas Rau, medical director of the Paracelsus Clinic in Lustmühle, Switzerland, have discovered the connection between *Candida* and mercury, postulating that one of the functions of the fungus in the body is to deal with heavy metals such as mercury, for which it has a particular affinity. If there is a high level of mercury in the body, *Candida* multiplies. Until you detoxify the body of the mercury, says Dr. Rau, you won't be able to get rid of the *Candida* overgrowth on any lasting basis, no matter how perfect your diet or what antifungal drug or natural substance you take. The fungus will just keep coming back.[53]

In addition to the previously mentioned digestive factors, food allergies are an obvious source of digestive difficulties, as the body is unable to adequately break down the problem foods.

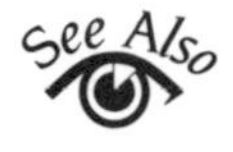

For information on the treatment of *Candida* overgrowth, see chapter 4.
For more about digestion and autism, see chapter 4; for allergies and autism, see chapters 4 and 5.

Allergies and Sensitivities

Just as autistic children may be hypersensitive to light, sound, or touch, they may also be hypersensitive to certain foods and food additives. Seeming allergies may actually be intolerances or sensitivities resulting from compromised immune and digestive systems. Once immunity is strengthened and digestive problems are eliminated or eased, the food intolerances may disappear. If unaddressed, the body's reaction to problem substances may be exacerbating or even causing the symptoms of autism. The autism-allergy connection is explored in depth in chapter 5.

It is important to consider here the concept of "brain allergies." Until recently, allergies were thought to affect only the mucous membranes, the respiratory tract, and the skin. A growing body of evidence indicates that an allergy can have profound effects on the brain and, as a result, behavior. An allergy or intolerance that affects the brain is known as a brain allergy or a cerebral allergy. The cases discussed in chapter 5 are examples of this type of allergic manifestation.

Dr. Rimland made the prediction at the 1972 annual meeting of the National Society for Autistic Children that "in 10 or 15 years the average physician will think of allergies as an immediate possibility when he sees an autistic-type child."[54] While this eventuality has not come to pass and many doctors continue to argue over whether brain allergies even exist, awareness of the issue is increasing in the medical profession.

Meanwhile, many parents of autistic children have discovered that they can produce significant improvement in their child's condition by removing problem substances from the diet. Mary Callahan, R.N., is one such parent. The author of *Fighting for Tony*, the story of her son's recovery from allergy-induced autism, Callahan appeared on national and local talk shows to try to get information about brain allergies to those who needed it most. "My goal is that someday the pediatric books will list allergy in the differential diagnosis of children with behavior disorders," she says.[55]

The substances that are frequently problematic in autistic children are gluten, casein, and food additives.

Allergy induced Autism (AiA), a group based in the United Kingdom, is dedicated to providing information on and increasing awareness of the connection between allergies and autism; visit their website at www.kessick.demon.co.uk/aia.htm.

Gluten and Casein

Gluten is a protein in wheat, barley, rye, oats, and other cereal grains. Casein is a protein in cow's milk and cow's milk products. During digestion, these large proteins (which are long chains of amino acids) are first broken down into smaller peptides before being further reduced into their amino acids

> **In Their Own Words**
>
> *"[Angela] would lie in her crib and stare at the ceiling or walls for long periods. If I called her name, she made no movement to come; she didn't even look up at me. If I interfered with what she was doing by picking her up, she would just stiffen and scream. . . . At three years old Angela was still totally non-verbal."*
>
> *After hearing about allergies that affect the brain, Donna took Angela, who by then had been diagnosed with autism, to a doctor who specialized in neurological allergies.*
>
> *"Now, one year later, Angela is a different child, as if she was never that bad and all the heart-ache was a collective nightmare for our family."*[56]
>
> —Donna Calvera,
> mother of Angela

components. Peptides are quite similar to endorphins in the brain, substances that serve as the body's natural painkillers and that athletes know as the source of "runner's high." The peptide forms of gluten and casein are called glutemorphins and casomorphins, respectively.

Researchers, beginning with Jaak Panksepp and others in the 1970s and continuing more recently with Paul Shattock and his colleagues, theorize that autism is caused by the incomplete digestion and subsequent excessive absorption of peptides from the intestines into the bloodstream.[57] The researchers hypothesize that the peptides travel into the brain across the blood-brain barrier. As glutemorphins and casomorphins are opioids, meaning they have an opium-like effect on brain cells, the effects are similar to those experienced by opium addicts: aloofness, irritability, insensitivity to pain, and stereotyped behaviors.[58]

Research has revealed higher than normal levels of urinary peptides in autistic children. Further, levels test closer to normal after children are put on a casein-free, gluten-free, or both casein- and gluten-free diet. Researchers also report that significant improvements in behavior and other areas accompany the dietary change.[59]

Foods That Contain Gluten

wheat
spelt
kamut
triticale
semolina
rye
oats
barley

Foods/Substances That Often Contain Gluten

vinegar
delicatessen meats
bouillon
dextrin
caramel color
food starch
hydrolyzed plant or vegetable protein
monosodium glutamate (MSG)
malt
rice syrup
natural and artificial flavorings

Foods/Substances That May Contain Gluten*

chewing gum
commercial spices
condiments
confectioner's sugar
envelope glue
frozen French fries
gravy
ice cream
instant coffee
ketchup
medications
mustard (vinegar)
Play-Doh
salad dressings
school glue/paste
tomato paste
tuna fish
vitamin/mineral supplements
yeast (packaged)

*Watch for hidden sources of gluten in the diet. Call the manufacturer of a product if you have any doubt.[60]

A long-term Norwegian study cited improvements in communication, social awareness, learning, problem solving, motor abilities, and bowel and bladder control, as well as reductions in emotional outbursts, resistance to change, avoidance of physical contact, stereotyped play, and odd body movements. In addition, autistic children who suffered from seizures had fewer episodes. The researchers stated that the remarkable improvements in the first year on the diet were not followed by regression, but by continued positive development over the next three years, although at a slower pace.[61]

For a comparison of results of removing wheat and dairy from the diet of autistic children, see the chart on page 39.

The Autism Network for Dietary Intervention (ANDI), established by parent researchers Karyn Seroussi (author of *Unraveling the Mystery of Autism and Pervasive Development Disorder: A Mother's Story of Research and Recovery*) and Lisa Lewis, provides information about gluten-free/casein-free diets. Contact ANDI at P.O. Box 17711, Rochester, NY 14617-0711 (fax: 609-737-8453) or visit their website (www.autismndi.com).

Food Additives

Sensitivity to food additives may reflect an already high toxic load and weakened immunity. Or there may be another reason why some autistic children do not seem to tolerate chemical additives. Such additives include: artificial flavoring, such as MSG; artificial preservatives, such as BHA, BHT, and TBHQ; artificial coloring/food dyes; thickeners; moisteners; and artificial sweeteners, such as aspartame. The more than 3,000 additives used in commercially prepared food have not been tested for their effects on the nervous system or on behavior.[62]

One double-blind, placebo-controlled study demonstrated that the ingestion of tartrazine (yellow dye #5) produced an increase in behavior problems in children sensitive to food coloring. The problems cited included crying, tantrums, irritability, restlessness, sleep disturbance, distractibility, and lack of control.[63] According to reports to the FDA (Food and Drug Administration), complaints associated with ingestion of aspartame include hypersensitivity to noise, ringing or buzzing in the ears, vision problems, gastrointestinal problems, irritability, and depression.[64]

According to the Feingold Association (the organization that arose out of the work of pediatrician and allergist Ben Feingold), cutting artificial additives out of the diet has been shown to be helpful for the following symptoms: hyperactivity, impulsivity, distractibility, short attention span, speech difficulties/delay, irritability, low tolerance for frustration, compulsiveness, perseveration, repetitive activity, frequent crying, sleep problems, ear infections, abnormal nystagmus, and hypersensitivity to touch, pain, sound, and light.[65]

Ben Feingold first introduced his findings about food additives at an American Medical Association meeting in 1973, reporting that additives were the source of the hyperactivity in 40 to 50 percent of the hyperactive children he saw as patients.[66] The Feingold diet, as the additive-free dietary plan is known, is controversial, in that a lot of effort has gone into debunking it. Dr. Rimland, in an article published in the *Journal of Learning Disabilities*, assessed the spate of research reviews that concluded that the Feingold diet was of little to no value.[67] He found serious flaws in their methodology and conclusions.

Again, as the controversy rages, parents of autistic children try the Feingold diet and find that it either helps their child or it doesn't. In data collected by the Autism Research Institute, of 527 cases of autism, 50 percent of the parents reported an improvement in their autistic child on the diet, while 48 percent said the diet had no effect, and 2 percent reported a worsening of behavior. (See the chart on page 39.)

The Feingold Association suggests that salicylate-containing foods may also be problematic for some children. Salicylates are natural compounds from which salicylic acid, the active compound in aspirin, is derived. Foods high in salicylates include strawberries and other berries, raisins, prunes, tomatoes, and nuts.

Salicylates are also added as flavoring to many commercially prepared sweet goods, such as cake mixes, puddings, licorice candy, chewing gum, and soft drinks.

For information about the Feingold diet, visit the website www.feingold.org or contact the Feingold Association in Riverhead, New York, at 516-369-9340.

Nutritional Deficiencies and Imbalances

Nutritional deficiencies and imbalances are another common feature of autism. Whether they are a contributing cause or a corollary of the disorder is unknown. Allergies, the limited range of foods characteristic of an autistic child's diet, and genetic factors may play a role in producing deficiencies. One imbalance often found in autistic individuals is a skewed copper to zinc ratio, with very high copper in relation to zinc. Chapter 6 discusses this imbalance as well as its probable cause.

Another common deficiency and imbalance is in essential fatty acids and the ratio of the different types. Supplementation may be beneficial in cases of autism. Supplementation with vitamin B_6 and magnesium in combination, vitamin A, or vitamin C may also be beneficial, indicating that deficiencies of these nutrients may be contributing to symptoms. (See the chart on page 39 for the results of supplementation with nutrients and other substances.)

Essential Fatty Acids

Research is uncovering a link between lipids and autism. Lipids are fats or oils, which are comprised of fatty acids. Examples of saturated fatty acids are animal fats and other fats, such as coconut oil, that are solid at room temperature. Examples of unsaturated fatty acids, which remain liquid at room temperature, are certain plant and fish oils. Essential fatty acids (EFAs) are unsaturated fats required for many metabolic actions in the body. There are two main types of EFAs: omega 3 and omega 6. The primary omega-3 EFAs are: ALA (alpha-linolenic acid); DHA (docosahexaenoic acid); and EPA (eicosapentaenoic acid). ALA is found in flaxseed and canola oils, pumpkins, walnuts, and soybeans, while DHA and EPA are found in the oils of cold-water fish such as salmon, cod, and mackerel.

Two important types of omega-6 EFAs are GLA (gamma-linolenic acid) and linoleic acid or cis-linoleic acid. Evening primrose, black currant, and borage oils are sources of GLA, while linoleic acid is found in most plants and vegetable oils, notably safflower, corn, peanut, and sesame oils. The body converts omega-3 and omega-6 EFAs into prostaglandins, which are hormone-like substances involved in many metabolic functions, including inflammatory processes.

The ratio of omega-3 to omega-6 EFAs is skewed in the standard American diet, which is deficient in omega 3s. High consumption of hydrogenated oils and beef contributes to the skewed ratio. Hydrogenated oils (which are oils processed to extend shelf life) are detrimental in two ways: not only does refining oil reduce its omega-3 content, but hydrogenated oils also interfere with normal fatty acid metabolism. Hydrogenated oils, also known as trans-fatty acids, are found in margarine, commercial baked goods, crackers, cookies, and other products. The problem with conventionally raised beef cattle is that they are grain-fed rather than grass-fed; grain is high in omega 6 and low in omega 3, while grass provides a more balanced ratio.[68]

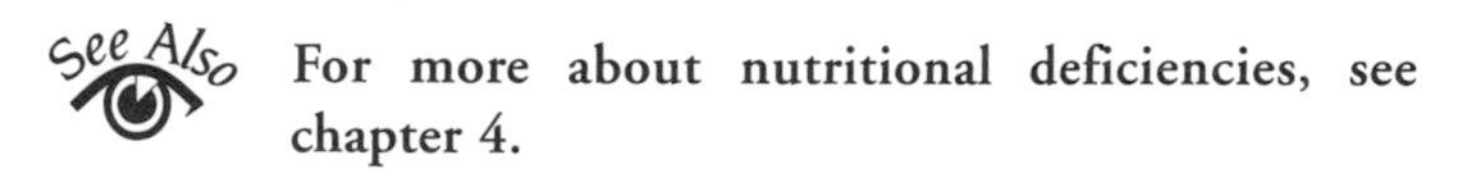

For more about nutritional deficiencies, see chapter 4.

Andrew Stoll, M.D., a psychopharmacology researcher and an assistant professor of psychiatry at Harvard Medical School, states: "Omega-3 fatty acids . . . are essential nutrients for human brain development and general health. Over the past 50 to 100 years, there has been an accelerated deficiency of omega-3 fatty acids in most Western countries. There is emerging evidence that this progressive omega-3 deficiency is responsible, at least in part, for the rise in the incidence of heart disease, asthma, major depression, bipolar disorder, and perhaps autism."[69]

Lipids are necessary for the health of the blood vessels that feed the brain and comprise 50 to 60 percent of the brain's solid matter.[70]

Andrew Stoll, M.D., a psychopharmacology researcher and an assistant professor of psychiatry at Harvard Medical School, states: "There is emerging evidence that this progressive omega-3 deficiency is responsible, at least in part, for the rise in the incidence of heart disease, asthma, major depression, bipolar disorder, and perhaps autism."

More specifically, nerve cells in the brain contain high levels of omega-3 fatty acids.[71] A deficiency, especially in a developing brain, could obviously have serious consequences.

Patricia Kane, Ph.D., founder of BodyBio, a medical research center in Millville, New Jersey, is one of the researchers who has been instrumental in calling attention to the role of lipids in autism. She states: "The level of fatty acids in the autistic child is an important factor because the endocrine system and its hormones, the brain and its neurotransmitters, and all the immune system components are derived from lipids. . . . The body requires specific fatty acids for the smooth running of the gastrointestinal system, the formation of cell membranes, nerve sheaths, and hormones, and for balance in the nervous system."[72]

Dr. Kane is a firm believer in blood chemistry analysis to determine the precise levels of an individual's nutrients. In this way, therapeutic intervention can be tailored to the precise needs.

Dr. Kane notes the further importance of this approach in relation to antioxidants (substances that protect cells from free radical damage), which include vitamins A, C, and E. "If you give antioxidants to autistic children, you may make them sicker," she states. "Their lipid disturbance is very different from that of a person with cardiovascular problems, for example, for whom taking antioxidants is a good idea. Children with autism require nutrients that *stimulate* oxidation, rather than prevent it, as antioxidants do; this is why vitamin E often produces negative effects in such children."[73]

Vitamin B_6 and Magnesium

"There is no biological treatment for autism which is more strongly supported in the scientific literature than the use of high dosage vitamin B_6 (given along with normal supplements of magnesium)," states Dr. Rimland.[74]

He cites 18 studies, published in the period from 1965 to 1996, that clearly demonstrated benefits of high dose vitamin B_6 for approximately half of the autistic study subjects. Magnesium is included in the protocol because it enhances B_6 activity and helps prevent the magnesium deficiency that can result from high doses of B_6. Of the 18 studies, 11 were double-blind, placebo-crossover. The reported benefits were in both behavior and laboratory measures of brain waves and urinary constituents, notes Dr. Rimland.[75] Among the behavioral benefits of this protocol cited over the years of research are improvement in attentiveness, responsiveness, play, appetite, speech, verbalization, cooperation, sleeping, bladder control, and overall health, and reduction in moodiness, frustration, temper tantrums, hyperactivity, self-stimulation, and bizarre behavior.[76]

Despite the evidence, many medical professionals still insist that there is nothing to support the efficacy of vitamin B_6 and magnesium in the treatment of autism. "A recent NIMH [National Institute of Mental Health] booklet on autism makes the blatantly false statement that 'clinical studies of the vitamin (B_6) have been inconclusive,'" says Dr. Rimland. "Eighteen consecutive positive studies, including 11 double-blind, placebo crossovers, are 'inconclusive'!"[77]

The vitamin-mineral protocol has the additional advantage of being "exceptionally safe," according to Dr. Rimland.[78] Side effects are rare and minor. Some people report digestive upset, which generally disappears when the dosage is adjusted. In very rare cases, numbness and tingling in the hands and feet occur, which disappear when the supplements are discontinued.

DMG for Autism

Dimethyglycine (DMG) is a substance similar to B vitamins and is found in the same foods. In fact, the active component in DMG is calcium pangamate, which is also called vitamin B_{15} or pangamic acid. Vitamin B_{15} arrived on the U.S. market after Russian researchers reported significant advances in speech in 12 of 15 children with mental handicaps who prior to supplementation with B_{15} had not communicated with speech. Subsequent legal battles resulted in a ban on the use of the term *vitamin* B_{15}. DMG is perfectly legal, however, and is currently classified as a food rather than a vitamin. It is safe, nontoxic, and available in health food stores. While symptoms of DMG deficiency are not apparent, supplementation has shown benefit for some people with autism.

A Korean researcher reported the results of three months of DMG supplementation in 39 autistic children. Benefits such as improved speech, appetite, excretion, and cooperation were seen in 80 percent, or 31 of the children, while the remaining eight children showed no benefits. The researcher noted that, during the first two weeks, eight of the children had sleep problems and six became more active. His conclusion was that DMG has benefit for children with autism.[79]

After nearly 25 years of following the DMG-pangamic acid issue, Dr. Rimland stated, "I am now so firmly convinced that DMG is helpful to a substantial proportion of autistic children and adults that I have decided to 'go public' in the *Autism Research Review International*—to tell people about it freely and openly, so they may try it if they wish."[80]

An average daily dose of vitamin B_6 in this protocol is around 8 mg per pound of body weight, says Dr. Rimland. For example, for a 60-pound child, the daily dose would be 480 mg (rounding up to 500 mg makes dosing easy). Some children do fine on less, some require more. For magnesium, the daily dose is 3 to 4 mg per pound of body weight. Again, for the 60-pound child, this translates into a dose of 180 to 240 mg daily.[81]

Parent Ratings of Behavioral Effects of Nutrients and Diets

Since 1967 the Autism Research Institute has been collecting parent ratings of the usefulness of the many interventions tried on their autistic children. The following data have been collected from more than 18,500 parents who have completed ARI questionnaires designed to collect such information. For the purposes of the present table, the parents responses on a six-point scale have been combined into three categories: "made worse" (refers to behavior only; ratings 5 and 6), "no effect" (ratings 1 and 2), and "made better" (ratings 3 and 4).

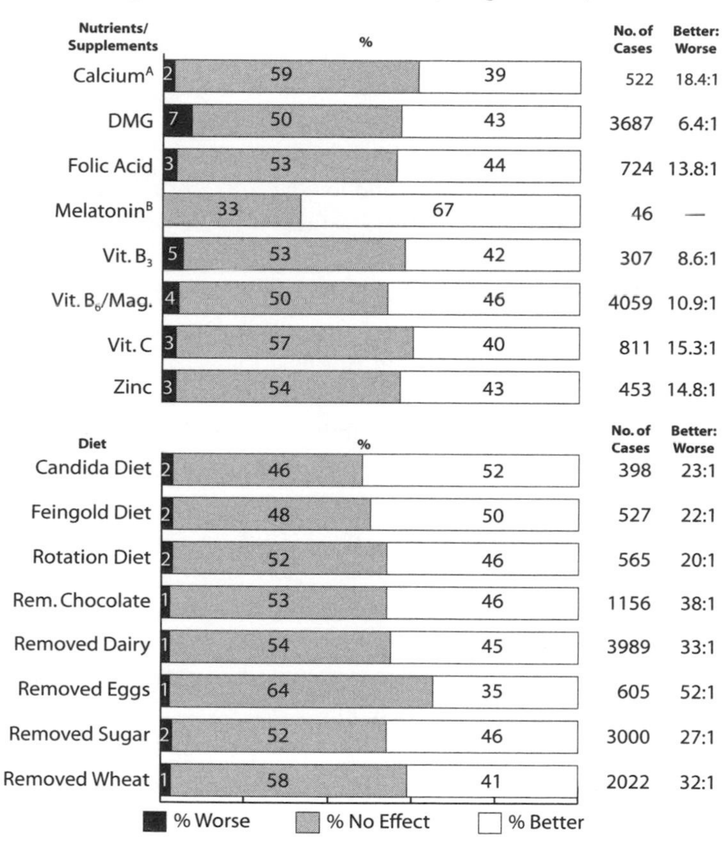

[A]Calcium effects not due to dairy-free diet; statistics similar for milk drinkers and non-milk drinkers.

[B]Caution: While melatonin can benefit sleep and behavior, its long-term effects on puberty are unknown.

Source: Adapted from ARI Publ. 34, September 2000. Reprinted by permission of the Autism Research Institute (4182 Adams Avenue, San Diego, CA 92116), 2002.

Dr. Rimland emphasizes, however, that "if extra B_6 helps an autistic child, it helps only because that child *requires* more B_6 than does a normal child. Of the various genetic neurological conditions which require large amounts of vitamins, B_6 is the vitamin most often required in massive amounts."[82]

Vitamin A

Researcher Mary Megson, M.D., a developmental pediatrician at the Pediatric and Adolescent Ability Center in Richmond, Virginia, has discovered that vitamin A may be deficient in children with autism for several reasons.[83]

First, they may not be able to absorb the form of vitamin A they are getting in their diets, which is typically vitamin A palmitate (found in infant formula and low-fat milk, for example). The mucosal lining of the intestinal tract needs to be healthy in order to absorb this form of vitamin A. As noted above, many autistic children have intestinal dysfunction and pathology.

Second, they typically are not getting sufficient dietary amounts of natural, unsaturated vitamin A, called the cis form of vitamin A, which can be absorbed even when the mucosal lining is damaged. The cis form is found in milk fat, liver, kidney, and cold water fish such as salmon or cod. Third, autistic children may have a defect in what is called G-alpha protein.

Dr. Megson suggests that the pertussis virus in the DPT (diphtheria-pertussis-tetanus) vaccine introduces a G-alpha protein defect in genetically susceptible children, and the measles virus vaccine depletes the child of vitamin A. Retinoid receptors, which moderate sensory input, require both G-alpha protein and vitamin A for their proper function. Retinoid receptors are critical for language processing, sensory perception, attention, and vision, explains Dr. Megson. She suggests that supplementation with the cis form of vitamin A may reconnect the receptors.

In a study of 60 autistic children, supplementation with cod liver oil (cis form of A), followed by Urocholine (a substance that stimulates receptors of the neurotransmitter acetylcholine) to address neurotransmitter dysfunction caused by blockage of G-alpha pathways, resulted in "dramatic, immediate improvements in language, vision, attention, and social interaction in some of these children . . . ," Dr. Megson reports.[84]

Improved eye contact, socializing, speech, toilet training, and sleep were among the specific benefits of the protocol.[85]

Vitamin C

Research suggests that vitamin C (ascorbic acid) may block dopamine receptors in the brain and produce a reduction in symptom severity when administered as a supplemental treatment in autism.[86] Dopamine is a neurotransmitter implicated in some psychoses and disorders involving abnormal movement. (Note that neuroleptic drugs such as Haldol, used with some autistic patients, block dopamine receptors.) One 30-week, double-blind, placebo-controlled study of 18 autistic people revealed that high doses of ascorbic acid reduced abnormal sensory-motor activity.[87] In some cases, nutritional testing of autistic patients reveals deficiencies in vitamin C (see chapter 4).

3 The Vaccine and Mercury Controversy

If vaccines are a causal factor in autism, why don't all children who are inoculated become autistic? This is a rhetorical question commonly raised as supposed evidence that vaccines can't play a role in the development of autism. The question is rendered pointless when you know the facts. If autism is a genetic disorder triggered by environmental factors, probably in combination, then there are multiple systemic weaknesses that make vaccines a hazard for vulnerable children, while children without these underlying conditions survive vaccination without apparent effect. (See chapter 7 for a discussion of the negative effects of vaccination on the immune system of even healthy children.)

The role of vaccines, along with the mercury many contain as a preservative, in the development of autism is perhaps the most controversial issue in the field today. In reviewing the literature, it seems evident that there is at least reasonable doubt regarding the safety of certain vaccines. Why then are they not pulled off the market while further study is undertaken? When you consider the stakes involved, the answer becomes clear—and it has a dollar sign in front of it.

More than 10 million vaccinations are given every year in the United States to children less than one year old, usually between two and six months of age.[88] The estimated global vaccine market for 2001 alone was $7 billion. According to the National Institutes of Health (NIH), there are currently 21 vaccine manufacturers, 91 marketed vaccines, and 367 new vaccines under development and in clinical trials.[89] The money flows in other directions, too. Federal and state governments fund vaccine programs to the tune of hundreds of millions of dollars annually; $526,167,000 in federal funding in fiscal year 2000; $134,787,881 in vaccine state grants from 1995 to 2000.[90]

On the other side of the equation, the costs are high. The Vaccine Adverse Event Reporting System (VAERS), a joint program of the FDA and CDC, had received 112,699 vaccine adverse reaction reports as of May 5, 2000, including 16,905 deaths and permanent disabilities. These numbers reflect only a tiny fraction of the actual numbers. The FDA itself estimates that only 1 to 10 percent of vaccine reactions are reported.[91]

Although research has not definitively proven that vaccines and mercury can cause autism, there is compelling evidence that they play a significant role, as you will see in this chapter. "The link between vaccines and autism is far stronger than the medical establishment is willing to admit, and very careful and well-reasoned research is an urgent priority," states Dr. Bernard Rimland. He adds that "[a]sking the CDC to look into vaccine safety is like asking the fox to guard the chicken coop. The CDC has been adamantly opposed to considering the possibility that vaccines may play a role in the causation of autism."[92]

Given the potential for severe consequences to thousands of children, the burden of proof should be on the vaccine manufacturers and the government bodies that are mandating childhood immunization, instead of on the public. As Tim O'Shea, D.C., author of *The Sanctity of Human Blood: Vaccination Is Not Immunization*, states, "As a nation, as a government, and as parents, Americans should be very certain, beyond a reasonable doubt, that any substance being injected into an unformed little nervous system is absolutely safe and does no harm."[93]

Let's consider the evidence.

Vaccines

The name *vaccine* arose from the first vaccination—for cowpox in the late 1700s—and comes from *vacca*, Latin for *cow*. A

Symptoms of Post-Vaccination Syndrome

According to Dr. Tinus Smits, the following are symptoms of acute and chronic post-vaccination syndrome (PVS).[94] Note how many symptoms, especially in chronic PVS, are also associated with autism.

Acute PVS

fever
convulsions
absent-mindedness
encephalitis and/or meningitis
swelling around the inoculation site
whooping-type cough
bronchitis
pneumonia
diarrhea
excessive drowsiness
frequent and inconsolable crying
penetrating shrieking
fainting
shock
death

Chronic PVS

colds
amber or green phlegm
inflamed eyes
loss of eye contact
squinting
middle ear inflammation
bronchitis
expectoration
coughing
asthma
eczema
allergies
inflamed joints
tiredness/lack of vigor
excessive thirst
diabetes
diarrhea or constipation
headaches
sleep problems with periods of waking and crying
epilepsy
rigidity of the back
muscle cramps
light-headedness
lack of concentration
loss of memory
growth disturbances
lack of coordination
disturbed development
behavioral problems including fidgeting and aggressiveness
irritability
moodiness
confusion
loss of willpower
mental sluggishness

vaccine is a preparation of an attenuated (weakened) or inactivated (nonlive) bacteria, virus, or other germ associated with a specific illness. In theory, the injected vaccine prompts the immune system to develop antibodies to the foreign proteins of the microorganism, and thereafter, the antibodies recognize and neutralize the microorganisms whenever they are introduced into the body, thus creating immunity to the illness involved.

In practice, the vaccination policy as it is implemented in the developed world, and increasingly in other nations, is resulting in a rising incidence of what Dr. Timus Smits, a Dutch homeopathic physician and leading authority on vaccines and their effects, terms post-vaccination syndrome (PVS).

"The fact that someone has displayed no direct or acute reaction to a vaccination does not necessarily exclude the possibility of the vaccine being the cause of chronic complaints," says Dr. Smits. "These complaints usually become clear only after one, two or even more weeks have passed and dismissing a diagnosis of PVS in chronic cases because of the time-lapse between the cause (vaccination) and the appearance of the condition is fundamentally wrong."[95]

A *Guide to Vaccines*

The National Vaccine Information Center (NVIC), a nonprofit educational organization working for the reform of the mass vaccination program, reports that vaccination rates for children under the age of three have risen from 60 to 80 percent of children getting DPT, polio, and measles vaccines in 1967 to 90 percent of children getting DPT, polio, MMR, and Hib vaccines in 1999.[96]

The following are the vaccines (with their abbreviated names) routinely given to children today:

DKTP: diphtheria-pertussis (whooping cough)-tetanus-polio
DPT/DTP: diphtheria-pertussis-tetanus
DTaP: diphtheria, tetanus, acellular pertussis
Hep B: hepatitis B

Hib: Haemophilus influenzae type B (this virus is a cause of meningitis in children)
MMR: measles-mumps-rubella
OPV: live virus oral polio
IPV: inactivated polio virus
Varicella: chickenpox

According to NVIC, in 1999, the average American child received the following vaccinations on the timetable cited. This adds up to 33 doses of 10 different viral and bacterial vaccines by the time the child is five years old:[97]

Hep B: at 12 hours of age and again at 1 month
DPT or DTaP, Hib, and OPV or IPV: at 2 and 4 months
DPT or DTaP, Hib, OPV or IPV, and Hep B: at 6 months
Live varicella: at 12 to 18 months
MMR and Hib: at 12 to 15 months
DPT or DTaP and OPV or IPV: at 18 months
DPT or DTaP, MMR, OPV or IPV: between 4 and 6 years.

Dr. O'Shea points to three particular days as "spectacularly toxic" for infants: shortly after birth when the baby receives the hepatitis B vaccine, which contains 12 mcg of mercury (30 times the official safe level); at 4 months when the infant receives the DTaP and HiB, with a total of 50 mcg of mercury (60 times the safe level), on the same day; and at 6 months when the child receives Hep B and polio on the same day, with 62.5 mcg of mercury (78 times the safe level).[98]

As noted in the previous chapter, the MMR vaccine seems to be particularly problematic for children who are susceptible to developing autism. In testimony before the U.S. Congressional Oversight Committee on Government Reform, Dr. Andrew Wakefield stated:

> "Rather than having parental reports alone of a temporal association between MMR exposure and developmental regression, there is now definitive evidence of a novel and

> specific pathology in the intestine of children with ASD [autistic spectrum disorder] that is associated with the presence of measles virus. In association with the findings of Kawashima et al., of measles virus in the peripheral blood of some children with ASD, it is no longer correct or acceptable to state that there is no evidence of an association between MMR and this syndrome. In light of this and in view of the acknowledged lack of adequate safety studies on the MMR vaccine, the case for making MMR vaccination either mandatory or the exclusive mode of protection against measles, mumps and rubella is, in my opinion, difficult to justify. Parents should be given an informed choice of vaccination strategy, including the provision of single vaccines."[99]

Dr. Wakefield's conclusions are supported by other medical professionals and researchers, who caution that focusing on the issue of removal of mercury preservatives from vaccines to the exclusion of other measures is not appropriate. (The MMR vaccine does not contain mercury.) Regardless of mercury, although that is doubtless an issue of vital concern, the viruses themselves in some cases are problematic, to say the least. Many people who have researched the subject believe that the number of different viruses given at one time is part of the reason for the great increase in autism.

The hepatitis B vaccine alone can have serious consequences, including death,[100] and the CDC policy of universal vaccination at birth has raised a public outcry. The policy is absurd, given that the avenues of contracting hepatitis B are, aside from being born to an infected mother, all far in the future for a new baby. Hepatitis B is spread by direct contact with infected bodily fluids, so the people at risk for the disease are IV drug users, prostitutes, prisoners, people with multiple sexual partners, and health-care workers.

Not only that, but there has been no long-term research into the side effects of the vaccine on infants, children, or adults, according to Bonnie Dunbar, Ph.D., a professor of molecular and cell biology at Baylor College of Medicine in Houston, Texas.[101] Worse, at the time that the universal vaccination mandate was announced, there were no peer-reviewed published studies demonstrating that the hepatitis B vaccine was safe to give to infants shortly after birth.[102]

As for the one place a baby could contract the virus, the incidence of mothers with the infection giving birth is far less than the five percent the CDC cited to justify universal hepatitis B vaccination. A 1999 study found that the incidence was actually only 0.2 percent, 25 times less than the CDC's claim.[103] In that same year, the CDC reversed its mandate for universal vaccination with hepatitis B and requested that drug companies manufacture a mercury-free hepatitis B vaccine, a move supported in a joint statement issued by the U.S. Public Health Service and the American Academy of Pediatrics.[104] Since then, such vaccines have arrived on the market, and newborns are routinely being vaccinated with hepatitis B again, although it is not mandatory.[105]

As with other environmental factors, sensitivity to vaccines, with or without mercury, may be the result of genetic weakness or the presence of a number of other factors that have left the system in a compromised state. An already weakened immune or nervous system will only be further weakened by vaccines, and the breakdown into autism may ensue. Although medical literature has documented vaccine-induced immune and brain dysfunction for more than 200 years, medical authorities still reject any link between vaccines and autism.

In 1991, with the pressure of ever greater numbers of parents reporting the regression of previously normal children into autism following DPT or MMR vaccination, the Institute of Medicine (IOM) published a report that stated that pertussis and rubella vaccines can indeed cause immune system and brain damage. Unfortunately, the IOM committee of physicians who then reviewed medical literature for evidence of the link rejected the initial conclusion, stating that no data identified a relationship between DPT vaccination and autism (MMR was not mentioned).[106]

Given the long-held view that autism is a psychological disorder, it is perhaps to be expected that there would be a paucity of research in this area. But a stronger factor may be the enormous pressure that is brought to bear when researchers publish findings that even suggest there may be a connection between vaccines and autism. Witness the attempts to discredit Dr. Andrew Wakefield. Virulent attacks on his integrity, professionalism, and medical expertise occurred after the publication of his article in the *Lancet,* as discussed in chapter 2. It is amazing that the measured, scholarly content and careful conclusions of this article produced such a reaction. Nowhere in the article does Dr. Wakefield say that measles vaccination causes autism. He simply suggests that further research is warranted.

Parents who are concerned about the vaccination issue may want to read this article, along with Dr. Wakefield's testimony before Congress, to draw their own conclusions about his findings. (See A. J. Wakefield, et al., "Ileal-lymphoid-nodular hyperplasia, non-specific colitis, and pervasive developmental disorder in children," *Lancet* 351 [February 28, 1998]: 637-41; and Andrew J. Wakefield, "Testimony to the Congressional Oversight Committee on Government Reform," available on the Internet at http://www.house.gov/reform/hearings/healthcare/01.04.25/wakefield.htm.)

The Hidden Ingredients in Vaccines

In addition to viruses and mercury, there are other substances that many vaccines contain that contribute to their toxicity. Most people are not aware that the vaccine their child is getting contains formaldehyde or MSG or any number of undesirable substances. The following are some of the ingredients used in the manufacture of a variety of vaccines:[107]

- Aluminum: suspected by the Environmental Defense Fund (EDF) to be a neurotoxicant, respiratory toxicant, cardiovascular or blood toxicant
- Ammonium sulfate: EDF-suspected neurotoxicant, respiratory toxicant, gastrointestinal or liver toxicant
- Amphotericin B: an antifungal drug with side effects that include blood clots, blood defects, kidney problems, nausea, fever, and potential allergic reactions

- Antibiotics (gentamicin sulfate, neomycin, polymyxin, streptomycin)
- Beta-propiolactone (chemical): EDF-recognized carcinogenic, EDF-suspected skin or sense organ toxicant, respiratory toxicant, gastrointestinal or liver toxicant
- Formaldehyde: EDF-recognized carcinogen, EDF-suspected neurotoxicant and immunotoxicant
- Hydrolyzed gelatin: derived from pieces of calf and cattle skins, demineralized cattle bones, and pork skin
- Monosodium glutamate (MSG): Concerns raised by the American Academy of Pediatrics resulted in the removal of MSG from products for infants under one year old; despite this, MSG is still in many (some say all) vaccines, even if the product insert does not list it.
- Phenol (carbolic acid): EDF-suspected neurotoxicant, developmental toxicant, skin or sense organ toxicant, respiratory toxicant, gastrointestinal or liver toxicant, kidney toxicant, cardiovascular or blood toxicant
- Phenoxyethanol (antifreeze): EDF-suspected developmental toxicant
- Polysorbate: EDF-suspected skin or sense organ toxicant
- Sorbitol: EDF-suspected gastrointestinal or liver toxicant
- Sucrose: refined sugar
- Thimerosal (methyl mercury): EDF-recognized developmental toxicant, EDF-suspected skin or sense organ toxicant
- Tri(n)butylphosphate (chemical): EDF-suspected neurotoxicant, kidney toxicant

Further, some manufacturers use material from cows (blood, fetal calf serum, meat broth) from countries that the U.S. government cites as having a risk of mad cow disease.[108] There are currently nine vaccines on the market containing such material.[109]

The following are examples of specific vaccines with some of the ingredients prominent manufacturers use to produce them:

- DtaP: formaldehyde, thimerosal, aluminum hydroxide, aluminum phosphate, polysorbate, gelatin
- DPT: aluminum phosphate, formaldehyde, ammonium sulfate, washed sheep red blood cells, thimerosal
- Hep B: aluminum hydroxide, thimerosal
- HIB: ammonium sulfate, formalin (formaldehyde solution), sucrose, thimerosal
- IPV: formaldehyde, phenoxyethanol, neomycin, streptomycin, polymyxin
- Live measles virus: neomycin, sorbitol, hydrolized gelatin
- MMR: sorbitol, neomycin, hydrolyzed gelatin

More Vaccines, More Autism

When you analyze the correlation between inoculation patterns and the enormous increase in autism, a connection is hard to refute. The number of autistic children, both in the U.S. and the U.K., rose precipitously after the introduction of the MMR combination, in 1978 in the U.S. and 1988 in the U.K. (see figure 3.1). The ten-year lag in the dramatic increase of cases in the two countries mirrors the ten-year difference in the introduction of the vaccine. Figure 3.2 depicts the correlation between the rise in autism and the increase in the number of doses and kinds of vaccines a child receives in the first two years of life.

Adverse Events Statistics

Vaccine Adverse Event Reporting System (VAERS) reports from January 1, 1990, to March 6, 2001, show the following statistics of adverse "events" following a selection of vaccinations.[110] VAERS is careful to state that the data contains "coincidental events and those truly caused by vaccines."[111] That's a lot of coincidence. And keep in mind that these are only the *reported* incidents, a very low percentage of the actual figures, as noted earlier.

	Adverse Events	Serious Adverse Events	Reported Deaths
DTP	21,163	3,286	794
HIB	21,726	3,905	932
MMR	20,974	2,586	132
Varicella (licensed in 1995)	12,635	590	31
Hep B	32,209	4,676	662

The following are useful resources for information on vaccines:

National Vaccine Information Center (NVIC)
421-E Church Street
Vienna, VA 22180
Phone: 703-938-DPT3
Fax: 703-938-5768
E-mail:
info@909shot.com
Website:
www.909shot.com

Illinois Vaccine Awareness Coalition (IVAC)
P.O. Box 946
Oak Park, IL 60303
Phone: 708-848-0116
E-mail:
info@vaccineawareness.org
Website:
www.vaccineawareness.org

PROVE (Parents Requesting Open Vaccine Education):
www.vaccineinfo.net

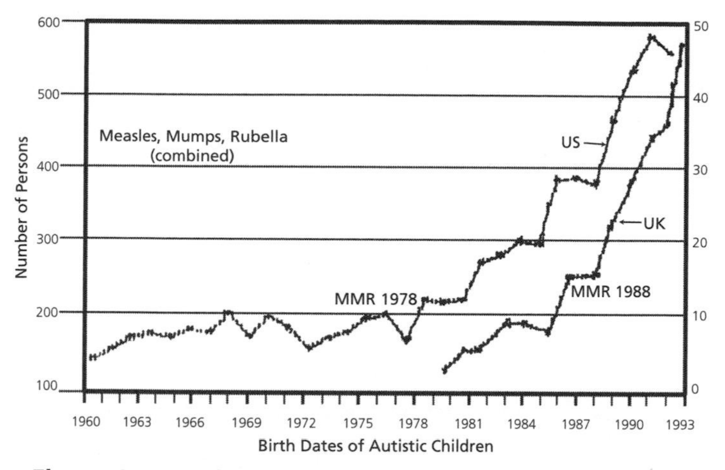

Figure 3.1. Autism Increase in U.S. and U.K. (10-year lag, 10-year difference in MMR introduction)

Source: Reprinted by permission of the Autism Research Institute (4182 Adams Avenue, San Diego, CA 92116), 2002; data from the California Department of Developmental Services.

F. Edward Yabak, M.D., a pediatrician and school physician who is now conducting research on vaccination, states, "The thing that increased at the same time as autism rates is vaccination. We now have the most vaccinated group of children ever. More importantly, the mothers of these children are also the most vaccinated mothers ever and have the most immune diseases ever in the history of the world."[112]

Safety Measures

Although there are safe alternatives to vaccines (see chapter 7), there are also measures that can be taken to reduce the potential effects of vaccination. To make the current immunization policy safer for the public, Dr. Tinus Smits has the following recommendations:[113]

1. Give vaccinations later. For example, in Japan, the whooping cough (pertussis) vaccination is not given until the child is two years old. (Dr. Smits notes that sudden infant death syndrome has become virtually nonexistent in Japan since implementation

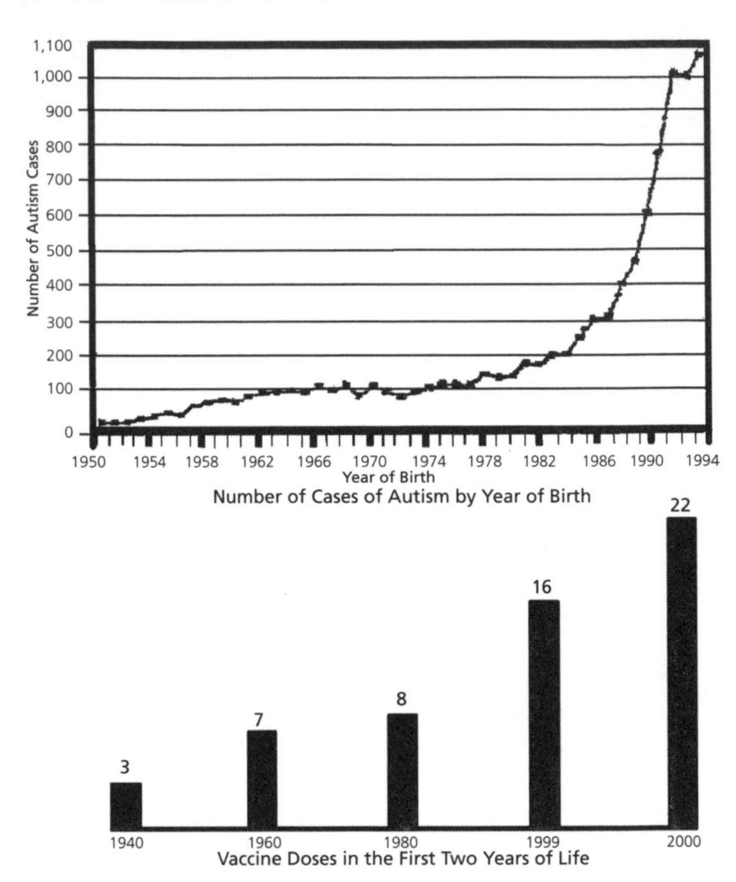

Figure 3.2. Cause or Coincidence?

Source: Reprinted from *Autism Research Review International* 14:4 (2000), by permission of the Autism Research Institute (4182 Adams Avenue, San Diego, CA 92116), 2002; data from the California Department of Health Services.

of this policy.) Waiting until then allows the child's immune system to mature and build up its general defenses.

2. Give vaccines separately where possible. In particular, never combine DKTP or DTP with the MMR.

3. Allow more time between vaccines: two months rather than one month.

4. Implement a "more stringent and cautious policy" than the current one regarding complications. This means keeping a careful record of a child's reactions to a vaccine and not giving the next vaccine until it is clear there are no complications.

5. Do not administer any more vaccinations until the child has recovered completely from post-vaccination symptoms.

6. Doctors, nurses, and parents need to be educated about post-vaccination syndrome.

While school districts across the country require children to be vaccinated with a variety of vaccines before starting school, parents should know that there are exemptions, depending on the state. Most states recognize medical or religious exemptions, while some grant exemptions on philosophical grounds as well.

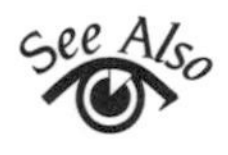

The majority of the chapters in part II of the book have information about vaccines and/or heavy metals such as mercury.

Mercury

The heavy metal mercury is well-recognized as a neurotoxin, and has been for centuries. Early hatmakers contracted what was known as "mad hatter's disease," the result of poisoning from the mercury used in hatmaking, hence the saying, "mad as a hatter." Physiologically, mercury's effects on the brain arise from its ability to bond firmly with structures in the nervous system, explains Dr. Dietrich Klinghardt, whose work is featured in chapter 11. Research shows that it is taken up in the peripheral nervous system by all nerve endings (in the tongue, lungs, intestines, and connective tissue, for example) and then transported quickly via nerves to the spinal cord and brainstem.

"Once mercury has traveled up the axon, the nerve cell is impaired in its ability to detoxify itself and in its ability to nurture itself," says Dr. Klinghardt. "The cell becomes toxic and dies—or lives in a state of chronic malnutrition. . . . A multitude of illnesses, usually associated with neurological symptoms, results."[114]

The use of thimerosal (methyl mercury) as a preservative in vaccines dates from the 1930s.[115] As noted earlier in the chapter, vaccines are now a major source of mercury for children within their first two years, partly due to the increased numbers of vaccines children receive. Thimerosal is employed as a preservative in nonlive vaccines, which include hepatitis B, DPT, DTaP, and Hib. (Live vaccines such as MMR and chicken pox do not contain thimerosal.)

Children who are susceptible to autism may have a compromised liver detoxification system, so their bodies are not able to get rid of the mercury as those without this defect may be able to do. This offers further explanation as to why some children are severely affected by vaccination and others are not.

As discussed in chapter 2, children who are susceptible to autism may have a compromised liver detoxification system, so their bodies are not able to get rid of the mercury as those without this defect may be able to do. This offers further explanation as to why some children are severely affected by vaccination and others are not. There is also a metal metabolism defect, often present in autism (this is explored at length in chapter 6), that makes mercury especially toxic for autistic children. Even with a normal system, an infant can't handle mercury. Bile is needed for the process of eliminating mercury from the body, but an infant's liver does not produce bile. The hepatitis B vaccine with its load of mercury is given to children before they have bile.

When you compare the manifestations of mercury poisoning and autism, the correspondence is startling. The sidebar on pages 58–59 shows that they are identical in many areas. Albert Enayati, a chemist and president of the New Jersey chapter of the Cure Autism Now Foundation (CAN), states, "As a trained scientist, my reading of the mercury literature indicates that every trait that defines autism can be induced by organic mercury."[116]

In addition to the mercury they get in vaccines, infants may be exposed to mercury before they are even born. Their mothers may be carrying a toxic load accumulated from mercury dental fillings (so-called silver fillings are actually comprised of more than 50 percent mercury), inoculations, and/or fish in the diet. The Environmental Protection Agency (EPA) estimates that 1.16 million women of child-bearing age in the United States eat enough mercury-contaminated fish to risk damage to the developing brains of any children they bear.[117]

The CDC stated in a report on its first study of mercury in human blood that even children of women who do not eat much fish may be at risk for the learning and intelligence disabilities associated with mercury poisoning.[118] The data reveal that the mercury problem is much larger than government agencies suspected. The report states that as many as 380,000 infants every year may be born to women exposed to mercury and be at risk for neurological disorders. Developing fetuses, and their nervous systems in particular, are especially vulnerable to the effects of mercury.

According to the FDA and the American Academy of Pediatrics (AAP), the amount of mercury infants get from immunizations has exceeded safety levels on both an individual and cumulative vaccine basis.[119] On May 31, 2000, the FDA informed vaccine manufacturers that reducing or eliminating thimerosal from vaccines was merited. Congressman Daniel Burton (R-Indiana), who has been pushing for changes in the current vaccine policy, states, "One would think that the FDA would have moved aggressively to remove vaccines that contained mercury from the market immediately. They did not. . . . The FDA continues to allow the mercury-containing vaccines to remain on the market. Today, over 8,000 children in America may be given a toxic dose of mercury in their vaccines."[120]

He also asks the pointed question: "How is it that mercury is not safe for food additives and OTC [over-the-counter] drug products, but it is safe in our vaccines and dental amalgams?"[121] Burton has a previously healthy grandson who developed autism after being inoculated with nine different vaccines in one day.

Summary Comparison of Traits of Autism and Mercury Poisoning

The following traits are all associated with both autism and mercury poisoning, as documented by researcher Sallie Bernard and colleagues, except where noted HgP stands for mercury poisoning and ASD for autistic spectrum disorder.

Psychiatric Disturbances

Social deficits, shyness, social withdrawal

Repetitive, perseverative, stereotypic behaviors; obsessive-compulsive tendencies

Depression/depressive traits, mood swings, flat affect; impaired face recognition

Anxiety; schizoid tendencies; irrational fears

Irritability, aggression, temper tantrums

Lacks eye contact; impaired visual fixation (HgP)/problems in joint attention (ASD)

Speech and Language Deficits

Loss of speech, delayed language, failure to develop speech

Dysarthria; articulation problems

Speech comprehension deficits

Verbalizing and word retrieval problems (HgP); echolalia, word use and pragmatic errors (ASD)

Sensory Abnormalities

Abnormal sensation in mouth and extremities

Sound sensitivity; mild to profound hearing loss

Abnormal touch sensations; touch aversion

Oversensitivity to light; blurred vision

Motor Disorders

Flapping, myoclonal jerks, choreiform movements, circling, rocking, toe walking, unusual postures

Deficits in eye-hand coordination; limb apraxia; intention tremors (HgP)/problems with intentional movement or imitation (ASD)

Abnormal gait and posture, clumsiness and incoordination; difficulties sitting, lying, crawling, and walking; problem on one side of body

Cognitive Impairments

Poor concentration, attention, response inhibition (HgP)/shifting attention (ASD)

Uneven performance on IQ subtests; verbal IQ higher than performance IQ

Poor short-term, verbal, and auditory memory

Borderline intelligence, mental retardation—some cases reversible

Poor visual and perceptual motor skills; impairment in simple reaction time (HgP)/ lower performance on timed tests (ASD)

Deficits in understanding abstract ideas and symbolism; degeneration of higher mental powers (HgP)/sequencing, planning, and organizing (ASD); difficulty carrying out complex commands

Unusual Behaviors

Self-injurious behavior (e.g., head banging)

ADHD traits

Agitation, unprovoked crying, grimacing, staring spells

Sleep difficulties

Physical Disturbances

Hyper- or hypotonia; abnormal reflexes; decreased muscle strength, especially upper body; incontinence; problems chewing, swallowing

Rashes, dermatitis, eczema, itching

Diarrhea, abdominal pain/discomfort, constipation, "colitis"

Anorexia; nausea (HgP)/vomiting (ASD); poor appetite (HgP)/ restricted diet (ASD)

Lesions of ileum and colon; increased gut permeability

Source: Reprinted by permission of Sallie Bernard, from S. Bernard, A. Enayati, L. Redwood, H. Roger, and T. Binstock, "Autism: A Novel Form of Mercury Poisoning," ARC Research, July 2000; available from ARC Research, 14 Commerce Drive, Cranford, NJ 07901 (tel: 908-276-6300); also available on the Internet at http://www.mercola.com/2000/oct/1/autism_mercury.htm

While the government drags its feet, the evidence linking thimerosal to autism is mounting. Researcher Boyd Haley, Ph.D., a chemistry professor at the University of Kentucky, states, "Thimerosal is extremely toxic. The preliminary data is convincing and does indicate that vaccines are the most likely suspect for causing autism."[122]

In October 2001, Andy Waters, of the law firm Waters and Kraus, announced that his firm had come into possession of a CDC confidential report on a study by CDC scientists investigating the link between autism and thimerosal in vaccines. (Waters and Kraus filed the first-known lawsuit alleging that thimerosal was responsible for the neurological damage in an infant later diagnosed with autism, and is currently heading a consortium of legal firms around the country who are representing similar cases.)

The CDC had previously released a version of the report that stated that the evidence was inconclusive. The confidential report, according to Waters, revealed quite different research results. For infants exposed to more than 62.5 mcg of mercury in their first three months, the study found that their risk of developing autism was 2.48 times more than the risk for infants who did not have that level of exposure.[123]

The lawsuits will likely help publicize this information and increase the growing pressure on the government to ban thimerosal-containing vaccines. The purpose of the legal action, says Waters, is "to bring to the surface the truth on this issue, a truth that government agencies seem unwilling to admit . . . , and to force the companies that profited from this disastrous mistake to shoulder the responsibility that so many families now bear on their own, often without even the aid of health insurance benefits."[124]

While it seems likely that the use of thimerosal as a preservative in vaccines will be phased out in the U.S., this is unfortunately not the case in developing countries. As a result of practical constraints and the high cost, it is not feasible there, according to the World Health Organization.[125] So vaccines will continue as a major source of mercury toxicity and potential neurological damage for children around the world.

Before turning to the natural medicine treatments that address vaccines, mercury toxicity, and other aspects of autism, I would like to note that the information presented in this chapter is only a small portion of the available data on the dangers of vaccines and mercury and their implication in the development of autism.

Part II

Natural Medicine Treatments for Autism

4 Targeted Therapeutic Nutrition and Heavy-Metal Detoxification

When Victoria George initially consulted clinical nutritionist Maile Pouls, Ph.D., about her six-year-old daughter, it was to see if Dr. Pouls could do anything to strengthen Hayley's immune system. For the previous two years, Hayley had contracted one illness after another, and been on antibiotics almost constantly. Recently, she had stopped eating and was so thin that her rib cage was visible. Doctors weren't offering real solutions and Victoria was afraid her daughter would have to be tube-fed. She was on the verge of checking her into the hospital when a friend told her about Dr. Pouls.

In the initial consultation, Dr. Pouls learned that Hayley was also autistic, and had a twin sister who was as well. Both girls typically had no affect, and would not look at their mother, interact, or be affectionate. They had never talked, and both engaged in the self-stimulatory behavior characteristic of autism. Hayley also displayed obsessive-compulsive behavior, endlessly switching light switches off and on. Both girls had evidenced developmental problems almost from the beginning, and were late in reaching all the usual markers, according to Victoria.

"Hayley didn't sit up until she was six months old, didn't walk until she was two years old, and, at six, she still wasn't speaking." Victoria wasn't seeking Dr. Pouls' help for her daughter's autism, however—because she didn't think help existed. Nothing had worked, and now her daughter was a picture of "failure to thrive."

Dr. Pouls, whose practice is based in Santa Cruz, California, proceeded with Hayley the way she does with all her patients. She ran a 24-hour urinalysis, which analyzes the total urine output of a 24-hour period, to get detailed information on Hayley's nutritional status and digestive competence, meaning how well she was digesting protein, carbohydrates, fats, and sugars (see sidebar on pages 68–69).

Based on the information from the urinalysis, Dr. Pouls then developed an individualized nutritional program for Hayley that included enzymes (the substances that break down food) to correct her particular digestive problems and supplements to redress her severe nutritional deficiencies. Dr. Pouls' treatment approach, which she calls Targeted Therapeutic Nutrition, is designed to improve digestion, remove stress factors, and deliver nutrients not only to reverse deficiencies, but also to support glands, organs, and systems.

"It was just phenomenal what happened," Dr. Pouls recalls. The wasting process was reversed, Hayley started gaining weight and building muscle, and her immune system rebounded, as evidenced by the fact that she stopped getting sick. But to Dr. Pouls, this was not the phenomenal part; she was used to seeing results like this with her treatment program. What was astonishing was that Hayley's autistic symptoms began to disappear. All of a sudden, after four months of treatment, she was smiling, interacting, and hugging her mother, her mental state obviously transformed. Her twin sister, who was not receiving treatment, remained the same as before.

What was astonishing was that Hayley's autistic symptoms began to disappear. All of a sudden, after four months of treatment, she was smiling, interacting, and hugging her mother, her mental state obviously transformed. Her twin sister, who was not receiving treatment, remained the same as before.

Prior to this, Dr. Pouls had had limited experience with autism, but she had witnessed many times the powerful effects of this relatively simple approach on all kinds of intractable health conditions. From her many years of experience, she knew the potential in identifying a person's nutritional, digestive, and toxic status and using enzymes, nutritional supplements, and detoxification protocols to rebalance their biochemistry.

After seeing the results with Hayley, Victoria brought her other daughter, Abra, to Dr. Pouls. "Abra's condition is more severe," states Victoria. Where Hayley was diagnosed with autistic spectrum disorder (ASD), Abra received no such softening of the autistic label. Abra was even more delayed than Hayley, says her mother, noting that Abra didn't walk until she was four. Unlike Hayley, she displayed aggressive behavior and suffered from a seizure disorder. She was on phenobarbitol for the seizures when Victoria took her to Dr. Pouls.

Abra's urinalysis report indicated more severe problems than Hayley's. While both twins showed a high degree of digestive incompetence, Abra's was more compromised and she tested severely deficient in calcium and vitamin C as well. Dr. Pouls started Abra on a program designed for her specific needs. This twin's response to treatment was similarly promising. "She came out of herself, and became interactive and affectionate," says Victoria, adding that Abra didn't have the mental jump that Hayley did, but the behavioral change was thrilling.

Upon seeing the initial startling results with Hayley, Dr. Pouls began to research autism and learned that heavy metal toxicity can play a role in the development of the disorder. Alerted to this problem,

The 24-Hour Urinalysis

Here are two urinalysis reports. The first is the initial 24-hour urinalysis Dr. Pouls ran on Hayley. The second was run after less than three months of treatment, and shows a significant improvement even in this short time. Following are explanations of what each value indicates and a comparison of Hayley's results.

Volume/Kidney Function: The total amount of urine produced in 24 hours, when compared to the specific gravity kidney concentration, reveals the state of kidney function. Hayley's function was normal in both tests.

Indican/Toxicity: Indican is a by-product of protein putrefaction in the large intestine when proteins are not properly broken down and so begin to rot. The higher the level of indican is, the greater the bowel toxicity. Hayley's first results showed severe bowel toxicity; her second, mild toxicity.

Calcium/Magnesium: This measures the levels of calcium and magnesium, which are necessary to support the skeletal, muscular, and nervous systems. Insufficient levels or an improper ratio between the two can produce anxiety, nervousness, hyperactivity, irritability, insomnia, muscle tension, spasms, cramps, low back pain, constipation, hypertension, or heart palpitations. In the first test, Hayley had very low magnesium and mildly low calcium; in the second, the levels of both were only slightly low.

pH: This measures the relative acidity or alkalinity of the urine on a scale of 0 to 14, with the acid values at the lower half of the scale and the alkaline at the upper half. Hayley showed excessive acidity in the first test; near normal values in the second.

Chloride Electrolytes: This is the amount of chloride (salt) residues in the urine, reflecting the body's assimilation of salt. It is also an indicator of trace mineral levels (assimilation). If chloride is low, trace minerals are generally low as well. Hayley's first test revealed an electrolyte/trace mineral deficiency; her values were normal in the second test.

Specific Gravity Kidney Concentration: This is the weight of substances dissolved in the urine (solutes) as compared to plain water. If the number is high, it means there are a lot of solutes in the urine, which indicates kidney stress. Hayley tested normal both times.

Sediment Nutrient Enzyme Reserve: This is a measure of the sediment (organic and mineral substances) in the urine after digestion. These sediments indicate undigested or poorly digested foods and attendant nutrient deficiencies. Hayley had poor digestion and absorption, indicating nutrient deficiency, in the first test; in the second test, she was upgraded to simply "poor utilization," with less nutrient deficiency.

Sediment Analysis: The three components of this analysis—calcium phosphate, uric acid, and calcium oxalate—indicate how well the body is digesting carbohydrates, proteins, and fats, respectively. The first test showed that Hayley had problems digesting all three food types; the second test showed improvement in her digestion of proteins and fats, while her difficulty digesting carbohydrates remained the same.

Vitamin C: This measures the body's vitamin C level. Vitamin C deficiency can result in lowered resistance to infections, impaired digestion, adrenal insufficiency, general weakness, and joint pain, among other conditions. Hayley's values were normal in both tests.

Non-Protein Nitrogen (NPN): This is a measure of protein metabolism, and indicates whether the body is in a state of anabolism (tissue building) or catabolism (muscle or tissue breakdown). Hayley's protein metabolism was normal in both tests.

Hayley's First Urinalysis Report

Volume/ Kidney Function	Indican/ Toxicity	Calcium Magnesium	pH	Chloride Electrolytes	SP Gravity Kidney Concentration	Sediment Nutrient Enzyme Reserve
Normal	3++	Light	5.9	05	1.017	1.10
Polyuria	4+		>8.0	>13	1.035	>1.2
2400 ml	2+	Milky	7.5	11	1.030	1.0
2000 ml	Trace	Heavy	7.0	09	1.025	0.7
1600 ml	Negative	Normal	6.5	07	1.020	0.5
1200 ml		Light	6.0	05	1.015	0.2
800 ml		Clear	5.5	03	1.010	Trace
Oliguria			5.0	01	1.005	None

Sediment Analysis			
Calcium Phosphate	Uric Acid	Calcium Oxalate	Vitamin C: 1 (normal: 1–5)
.30	.50	.30	Non-Protein N: 4 (normal: 3–5)

Hayley's Second Urinalysis Report

Volume/ Kidney Function	Indican/ Toxicity	Calcium Magnesium	pH	Chloride Electrolytes	SP Gravity Kidney Concentration	Sediment Nutrient Enzyme Reserve
Normal	2	Light/Nor	6.3	07	1.022	.80
Polyuria	4+		>8.0	>13	1.035	>1.2
2400 ml	2+	Milky	7.5	11	1.030	1.0
2000 ml	Trace	Heavy	7.0	09	1.025	0.7
1600 ml	Negative	Normal	6.5	07	1.020	0.5
1200 ml		Light	6.0	05	1.015	0.2
800 ml		Clear	5.5	03	1.010	Trace
Oliguria			5.0	01	1.005	None

Sediment Analysis			
Calcium Phosphate	Uric Acid	Calcium Oxalate	Vitamin C: 1 (normal: 1–5)
.30	.40	.20	Non-Protein N: 4 (normal: 3–5)

she ran a hair analysis on Hayley and later on Abra. Hayley's test indicated only slightly elevated levels of nickel and aluminum, and a normal lead level. Abra's hair analysis, however, revealed that she had a very high level of lead (1.10, with normal being 0-0.5) and a significantly elevated aluminum level (13.6, with normal at 0-8) as well. Victoria does not know for certain the source of Abra's lead exposure and why Hayley escaped the exposure and/or its effects, but she thinks it may be because "Abra mouths things a lot more. Maybe there was lead in the paint on some toys."

Dr. Pouls started Abra on an oral chelation product she had developed to rid the body of heavy metals such as mercury and lead because she had discovered that toxicity was a factor for many of her clients. In this therapy, a chelating agent binds (chelates) with the heavy metals and both are then excreted from the body.

With the chelation, Abra showed another level of improvement. "She was more aware and interactive, and her eye contact got better," says Victoria. Her aggressive behavior also decreased greatly. This may have been the result of removing the lead; numerous studies have established a link between high lead levels and aggression.

The twins continued on their supplement protocol and more improvements unfolded. "Within a year of beginning treatment, Hayley started talking," declares Victoria. "Actually, she started writing first, then talking." The self-stimulatory behavior ended, as did Hayley's obsessive-compulsive pursuits. Hayley's immune system and overall health are strong, and Abra was weaned off the phenobarbitol as her seizures stopped. With the recent return of mild seizures, Abra is back on a medication, but a less powerful one, while Victoria and Dr. Pouls continue to work on the problem nutritionally.

Both twins are still making gains in their development. Hayley is ahead of Abra, mentally and neurologically, notes Dr. Pouls, because she started treatment earlier and Abra's imbalances were more severe. Abra is still not talking, but she now goes to school, something she couldn't do before because of her aggression. Hayley is about two grade levels below others of her age, Victoria estimates, but she improved a grade level this past year. Both girls are in a special needs program within the public school, and Hayley has begun integration into the mainstream classroom.

"I have no doubt that she will go on to be a perfectly normal child and successful adult," states Victoria.

Victoria speaks of how Dr. Pouls' treatment released her daughters into their personalities, allowing them to be who they are instead of being ruled by their biochemical state. She wants all parents of autistic and other special needs children to be able to benefit from this type of treatment. With that in mind, she started a nonprofit organization called BALANCE (Bringing Alternative Learning and Nutritional Choices to Education) dedicated to "bringing alternative supplemental programs to public education."

> **In Their Own Words**
>
> *"I'm pretty convinced [Dr. Pouls'] regimen is what turned my daughters around. Hayley's been very balanced for the last year and a half, and she continues to improve. The fact that Abra's in class is just huge for me. Families with autistic children know how stressful it is. . . . My message to all parents is . . . have this testing to find out what is going on in the child. Address the imbalances and see what the effect is on behavior."*
>
> —Victoria George,
> mother of Hayley and Abra

She is working with her local school system to get information about nutritional treatment and other alternative therapies to those who need it. Further, in recognition of the lack of health coverage of many alternative therapies and the consequent expense involved, BALANCE plans to arrange donated therapies and fundraising for those who require financial assistance.

For information about BALANCE, see their website at www.balance4kids.org or call them in Santa Cruz, CA, at 831-464-8669.

Testing as the First Step in Treatment

Since Hayley began treatment, Dr. Pouls has worked with numerous children with autistic or behavioral disorders. "A lot of the parents who come to me are in the dark—and so are a lot of their health practitioners—as to what to do," comments Dr. Pouls. "Unfortunately, they're given drugs. That's the number one thing that's done for their children." Many of the children she sees have already been through a string of drugs, which not only haven't worked, but have also produced numerous side effects. "They're seriously nervous, fidgeting, have tremors, severe anxiety, fear, nightmares, and repetitious body movements. With the drugs, their symptoms often get worse."

"Many of the parents who come to me have no hope," she continues. "They don't even go to the place in their mind that this child could be functioning and back in the world." Dr. Pouls is here to tell parents that there is hope. "These children—that's the wonderful thing about children—respond very quickly," says Dr. Pouls. "The parents usually see changes in two to three weeks—significant changes in at least some of their problems or symptoms. Every child is different. I'd say there are some that are back to almost 100 percent. Then there are others that we've gotten back to 70 percent, but some of them have just started on the program."

She urges parents to find out what's actually happening in their child at a biochemical level. "It's crucial to do preliminary urine and hair analyses to measure a child's individual deficiencies. Some practitioners do too much all at once without knowing what's going on; they just start giving protocols and products without evaluating where the major issues are." This can be expensive, in terms of both money and the emotional and psychological costs to parent and child when the treatment doesn't work.

The majority of parents who come to Dr. Pouls have financial restraints, so she tries to be conservative in the amount of tests she runs and focuses on their highest treatment priorities. "For most children, I just do the hair analysis and the urinalysis. That's sufficient to show me the direction I need to take in treatment."

In addition to measuring the extent of heavy metal toxicity, hair analysis also shows the level of minerals that are crucial for brain cell function and overall health. The urinalysis not only pinpoints biochemical imbalances and nutritional deficiencies that directly affect the health of organs, glands, and systems, it also identifies digestive competence or incompetence, enzyme status and deficiencies, and certain organ stresses such as colon toxicity and liver toxicity.

Despite the far greater amount of information it provides, the 24-hour urinalysis Dr. Pouls runs is not the standard test used in most doctors' offices, clinics, and hospitals. For the standard test, the patient gives a single sample of urine, versus collecting all of the urine excreted over a 24-hour period. "The specific type of urine evaluation that I do is not done by many health-care providers," notes Dr. Pouls. "It's unfortunate that there are so few practitioners who understand the value of looking at underlying nutritional deficiencies and imbalances in relationship to symptoms." In addition, most laboratories don't do the 24-hour urinalysis.

Dr. Pouls uses the following laboratories for the tests discussed here: for 24-hour urinalysis, Metabolic Research Lab in Overland Park, KS (tel: 888-326-6367 or 913-345-0088); for elemental hair analysis, Great Smokies Diagnostic Laboratory in Asheville, NC (tel: 800-522-4762 or 828-253-0621; www.gsdl.com). This information may be helpful to your doctor.

After reviewing the results of the hair and urine analyses, Dr. Pouls initiates treatment based on what the tests reveal. With children who have autistic symptoms, she approaches treatment in two phases. The first focuses on correcting digestive problems and reversing nutritional deficiencies. Supplementation with natural products to support the liver, stengthening its detoxification abilities, is also often part of the initial phase. In some cases, the first phase is sufficient to restore the child to health. In other cases, the second phase of employing oral chelation to detoxify the body of heavy metals such as mercury and lead is necessary. Children respond fairly quickly to this type of treatment, notes

Dr. Pouls. "Usually, 60 to 90 percent of the shifts happen in the first two months."

Restoring Digestion

Many children labeled autistic or exhibiting autistic symptoms have digestive problems and tend to eat a limited range of foods. Whether due to nutrient absorption problems or to not eating enough nutrititious food, most have nutritional deficiencies. Dr. Pouls believes that the first order of treatment is to get these children's digestive systems working again, so their growing bodies can start getting the nutrients they desperately need. As discussed in chapter 2, food allergies or intolerances and fungal (*Candida*) overgrowth in the intestines are common digestive problems that need to be addressed. Supplementation with digestive enzymes and acidophilus is key here.

Children with autism frequently suffer from what are labeled food allergies, but Dr. Pouls states that the majority of these so-called allergies are not true allergies. Instead, they are food intolerances resulting largely from poor digestion. Often, when you correct the digestion, the sensitivity to various foods disappears.

Food Allergies/Intolerances

Children with autism frequently suffer from what are labeled food allergies, but Dr. Pouls states that the majority of these so-called allergies are not true allergies. Instead, they are food intolerances resulting largely from poor digestion. Often, when you correct the digestion, the sensitivity to various foods disappears.

Food intolerances occur when the body doesn't digest food adequately, which results in large undigested protein molecules entering the intestines from the stomach. When poor digestion is chronic, these large molecules push through the lining of the intestines, creating the condition known as leaky gut, and enter the bloodstream. There, these substances are out of context, not recognized as food molecules, and so are regarded as foreign invaders. The immune system sends an antibody (also called an immunoglobulin) to bind with the foreign protein (antigen), a process which produces the chemicals of allergic response. The antigen-antibody combination is known as a circulating immune complex, or CIC. Normally, a CIC is destroyed or removed from the body, but under conditions of weakened immunity, CICs tend to accumulate in the blood, putting the body on allergic alert, if you will. Thereafter, whenever the person eats the food in question, an allergic reaction follows.

Dr. Pouls estimates that at least 85 percent of what appear to be food allergies in autistic children are not true allergies. For this reason, she does not immediately run allergy testing to isolate potential food allergens (substances that produce an allergic reaction). The treatment response to such a test is to remove that food from the diet. As many children with autism are extremely finicky eaters and are already eating only a few foods, or they are already on a restricted diet due to previous doctors' recommendations, Dr. Pouls prefers to approach the problem in another way.

Rather than radically reducing a child's diet even further, she relies on a three-point treatment to deal with ostensible allergies: 1) using enzymes to improve digestion, which stops the reactions to foods that aren't real allergens but are presenting as such; 2) employing protease enzymes to clear the CICs

About Enzymes

Enzymes are special proteins that are involved in all chemical reactions in the body. That means they are essential for energy production and the normal function of everything from a single cell to a body-wide system. Enzymes are central to the digestion and absorption of food. Different types of enzymes break down different types of food, as follows: protease for proteins, amylase for carbohydrates, lipase for fats, cellulase for fiber, and disaccharidases for sugars.

out of the bloodstream, for the same reason and to lift a huge immune load off the child; and 3) healing the gut lining with specific nutrients to stop undigested food molecules from entering the bloodstream and perpetuating food intolerances or creating more of them.

We get our digestive enzymes from two sources: the pancreas manufactures them, and raw foods contain them. If we eat a diet of processed, refined foods, the pancreas has to supply all the enzymes needed for digestion. This places undue stress on that organ. If the diet is chronically enzyme-depleted, the pancreas cannot keep up with the demand for enzymes, and digestion and other body functions begin to suffer. Compromised immunity is one result because the immune system donates its enzymes to complete the digestive process, thus depleting its own supply.

The specific enzymes Dr. Pouls puts a child on depends upon the results of the urinalysis, which shows whether or not the patient is breaking down carbohydrates, proteins, and fats and to what degree. Dr. Pouls also uses the information provided by an in-depth food diary and food chart filled out by the parent. In revealing patterns in dietary reactions, these records can indicate food intolerances and their attendant enzyme deficiencies. For example, if a child gets diarrhea after eating eggs, he may have an "allergy" to eggs and/or a deficiency in protease (the enzyme that breaks down proteins). If the food reaction is due to poor digestion, supplementing with protease can correct that deficiency and enable him to digest eggs, thereby clearing up the food sensitivity. If he has a true allergy to eggs, protease supplementation can reduce the severity of the reaction.

In Dr. Pouls' experience, her three-point treatment approach successfully clears up "allergies" in most cases, and is far easier on both parent and child than the restrictive diets many doctors prescribe. "My approach may be more conservative than what a lot of health practitioners would require of these parents and children. But I find that with the steps I take, we get results and the compliance is better. If the treatment program is too difficult or too expensive, the follow-through will be poor," notes Dr. Pouls.

With her approach, it is rarely necessary to implement an extreme diet. "The parents are really overwhelmed," she adds. "I want to make it simpler for them, and more doable. My goal is to help the children to immediately start digesting and assimilating properly and get the most out of whatever they are willing or able to eat, with the least amount of reaction."

At the same time, however, Dr. Pouls suggests that parents gradually cut back on the major foods that most children are reactive to, those being dairy, sugar, chocolate, nuts (especially peanuts), wheat, and eggs. "I don't suggest cutting these out completely in the beginning," she says, "because these children have been so restricted for so long and some of them are so thin that if you remove those foods immediately, you're going to get a child going downhill." She does, however, highly recommend completely eliminating, if possible, foods containing preservatives and artificial sweeteners, flavoring, and coloring.

If people want to keep dairy in their diet, Dr. Pouls advocates using only organic dairy products. "Do you know that one pound of commercial butter may contain more residues of pesticides, herbicides, and chemicals than you get in eating a whole year's worth of commercial fruits and vegetables?" She notes that cattle in the commercial dairy industry are overloaded with chemicals. Their livers can't keep up with processing the toxins, so the toxins are stored in fat. "The highest concentration is found in butter, followed by cheese, then milk, then meat, in that order," says Dr. Pouls. "I tell my patients to buy organic dairy whenever possible."

The parents have options in their approach to diet, Dr. Pouls stresses. They can eliminate the top one or two foods, the foods the child reacts most strongly to, or they can cut back on those foods, and give the child double the appropriate enzyme when he eats the problem food. The latter minimizes the allergic reaction, explains Dr. Pouls. For instance, if a child is lactose intolerant, or allergic to dairy products, giving the child lactase when he eats dairy can reduce the effects. Or if he has a sugar intolerance, he can take sucrase when he eats something with sugar in it.

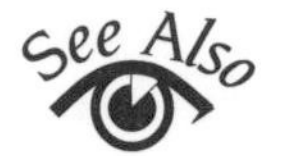

For more about allergy treatment, see chapter 5.

Following a rotation diet is another method that can allow the child to continue having foods she loves, even the highly problematic ones. The reason the child reacts more and more strongly to these foods is the huge CIC load in the bloodstream, which makes the body more reactive than it needs to be, explains Dr. Pouls. By only giving the food every four days, you allow the immune system to clear out the CICs and the body becomes less reactive.

Clearing the CICs from the bloodstream is the second point in Dr. Poul's three-point approach to reversing allergies. Giving the child protease enzymes between meals is an excellent means of accomplishing this, when combined with improving digestion and healing the gut to prevent further formation of CICs. "When taken on an empty stomach, protease is absorbed into the bloodstream where it acts like a scavenger, eating up CICs and other debris like a little Pac-Man," says Dr. Pouls.

If the parent wants to go further in investigating the child's food allergies and find out all the foods he is reactive to, Dr. Pouls relies on a sophisticated blood analysis, called the Food Antibody Assessment. Far superior to the old method of a separate pinprick on the arm for every single food tested with the accompanying wheal if the child is allergic, this involves one drawing of blood for a test of as many as 100 foods. It both identifies problem foods and rates the severity of reaction to each.

The Food Antibody Assessment and other allergy tests are available through Great Smokies Diagnostic Laboratory in Asheville, NC (tel: 800-522-4762 or 828-253-0621; www.gsdl.com). This information may be helpful to your doctor.

Enzyme Supplementation

Not only is supplementing with enzymes important in reversing food sensitivities, but it is also the quickest means of ensuring that the child is getting the greatest amount of nutrients from the limited food she is eating. With enzyme deficiencies, foods are not getting broken down adequately, and the nutrients they contain are therefore not being made available to the body. Further, undigested food putrefies and ferments, which disturbs the body's pH balance, tipping it into excess acidity.

Dr. Pouls notes that people often ask her how a child can become deficient in enzymes so quickly, meaning, already in the space of their short lives. Her answer is that they may have been born with a low enzyme reserve. In addition, a poor diet of mainly cooked and processed food can produce an enzyme deficiency relatively rapidly, as the pancreas is forced to keep up with the demand for enzymes, with no supply coming in from dietary sources.

So, as soon as possible, Dr. Pouls starts the child taking the enzymes he lacks as revealed by the urinalysis report. Most of the children with autistic symptoms that Dr. Pouls sees test very poorly on breaking down protein, which indicates protease enzyme deficiency. With this disability in breaking down proteins, many autistic children are severely deficient in amino acids (the components of protein). Among their many functions in the body, amino acids are needed for building muscle, tissue repair, formation of hormones and neurotransmitters, and immune activity. Decreased amino acids result in a decrease in calcium and magnesium because these minerals need to bind with amino acids for transport into tissues. Anxiety, nervousness, and hypersensitivity are some of the results of calcium and magnesium deficiency.

Amino acid deficiency has obvious implications, then, for growing children and for the common pattern of continual illnesses. Children under stress need even more amino acids than children leading a more placid existence. Certainly, autism is a stressful condition. In addition, poorly digested proteins place stress on the kidneys and liver. These organs are usually already taxed by toxins—the viral load from vaccines and heavy metals from vaccines, air, water, and food—associated with autism.

Supplementing with the enzyme protease (if the child doesn't have an irritated stomach lining) can ameliorate all of these problems by getting the digestion of protein going and the vital supply of amino acids flowing, while lifting some of the burden from the overworked liver and kidneys.

An added benefit of enzyme supplementation is that enzymes don't die and are not excreted. Instead, they work until they're exhausted. Taken with food, they help digest it, but if there are any enzymes left over, they are stored in the pancreas or other tissue for future use.

Fungal Overgrowth

Another common digestive problem among autistic children is intestinal overgrowth of the yeast-like fungus *Candida*. It is important to address this problem, states Dr. Pouls, because candidiasis (*Candida* overgrowth) contributes to the development of leaky gut syndrome, which permits those large undigested protein molecules to enter the bloodstream from the intestines and initiate the development of food allergies.

Many of the children Dr. Pouls treats are seriously immune-compromised, so they have had a string of illnesses and numerous courses of antibiotics, which kill the good bacteria as well as the bad, as explained in chapter 2. The lack of beneficial bacteria in the intestines is what allows the *Candida* normally present to run rampant. Intestinal dysbiosis (imbalance in intestinal flora) is the result. High mercury levels in the body also contribute to an overgrowth of *Candida*, she notes.

"I assume intestinal dysbiosis with almost all of the children who come to me with autistic symptoms," states Dr. Pouls. "If they've been on antibiotics, they probably have a complete depletion of acidophilus [beneficial intestinal bacteria]." Given that, Dr. Pouls has the children take a formula that contains a cellulase enzyme, which "eats" *Candida* and other fungus, and live culture, nondairy acidophilus to repopulate the intestines with the beneficial bacteria. With this formula, "you're killing the unhealthy flora, and replenishing with healthy flora," explains Dr. Pouls. Further, since the enzyme eats the yeast, it prevents the die-off side effects, which are often quite unpleasant, that people experience with other *Candida* protocol products. She notes, however, that as long as there are high levels of mercury in the body, *Candida* overgrowth will keep recurring.

Stool analysis is a simple means of determining the degree of intestinal dysbiosis. The test Dr. Pouls relies on identifies the level of *Candida* and other abnormal flora, as well as beneficial bacteria levels. It also determines whether parasites, amoebas, or worms are present. This is often the case when the immune system is compromised, as it is in autistic children, says Dr. Pouls. The test also pinpoints the degree of leaky gut or intestinal permeability.

Dr. Pouls doesn't automatically run the stool analysis, however. "I know it's a top priority with most of these children to start restoring the gut, so I usually just work initially on the *Candida,* without the additional expense of laboratory testing. Then I reevaluate to see if the stool analysis is necessary."

It is important to note that conventional antifungal medications often prescribed for autistic children with candidiasis do not address the underlying factors that allowed the fungal overgrowth in the first place. Without correcting these factors, lasting and comprehensive health benefits are unlikely. As biochemist and autism authority William Shaw, Ph.D., notes, "Even after six months, and sometimes even after two or three years, of antifungal treatment [drug therapy], there is often a . . . loss of improvements after discontinuing antifungal therapy."[126]

The Comprehensive Digestive Stool Analysis/ParasitologyX3 is available through Great Smokies Diagnostic Laboratory in Asheville, NC (tel: 800-522-4762 or 828-253-0621; www.gsdl.com). This information may be helpful to your doctor.

Healing the Gut

The cellulase-acidophilus formula won't heal the gut lining; it only gets rid of the culprit (*Candida*), says Dr. Pouls. To reestablish the integrity of the intestinal lining, a necessary step in restoring digestion to optimum function, she uses nutrients and herbs known to aid in rebuilding it. These include:

- L-glutamine: an amino acid that supports the growth and function of the mucous membrane lining the gastrointestinal tract[127]

- N-acetyl-glucosamine (NAG): a form of glucosamine, a substance that aids in cartilage repair in joints; NAG is a precursor needed for production of glycoproteins, which form a protective layer in the intestinal mucosa[128]

- gamma-linolenic acid (GLA): an omega-6 essential fatty acid found in high concentrations in borage seed oil; GLA is a precursor of the anti-inflammatory prostaglandins[129]

- gamma oryzanol: a component of rice oil with therapeutic effects on gastrointestinal disorders[130]

- slippery elm (*Ulmus rubra, U. fulva*): a demulcent (rich in mucilage) herb known for its ability to soothe and protect inflamed mucous membranes in the digestive tract.[131]

Nutritional Deficiencies

With digestion improved and enzyme supplements ensuring assimilation of nutrients, supplementation with vitamins, minerals, and other nutrients that the 24-hour urinalysis and hair analysis (for minerals) have revealed the child to be deficient in can be implemented. It is important, according to Dr. Pouls (and many other natural medicine practitioners), to rebuild the digestive system first, otherwise it is likely that the body won't be able to absorb the supplements.

As previously noted, many children with autistic symptoms are severely deficient in amino acids. Almost all of those Dr. Pouls treats require amino acid supplements. She uses organic, plant-based amino acids that are already broken down for easy digestion.

She has also found that almost all of the children are severely deficient in minerals and electrolytes. (The 24-hour urinalysis shows deficiencies in major minerals such as calcium and magnesium, while hair analysis picks up deficiencies in trace minerals, such as zinc.) As minerals are essential for brain cell, nerve cell, and muscular function, such deficiencies have a profound impact. "Every cell of the body needs electrolytes and trace minerals," states Dr. Pouls. "Sometimes, by giving a child liquid ionic minerals, just that alone, they'll notice a positive shift." Further, supplementation with ionic minerals alkalinizes the system, helping to reverse an overacid pH.

Although many forms of minerals are available, liquid ionic minerals are a highly absorbable form. "I have found that ionic minerals are the kind that are most easily used by the body for nutrient transport and waste removal from the cells (ionic transport)," she says, adding that the evidence for this is in the urinalysis results.

Many children with autistic symptoms are severely deficient in amino acids. Almost all of those Dr. Pouls treats require amino acid supplements. She uses organic, plant-based amino acids that are already broken down for easy digestion.

The most severe mineral deficiencies Dr. Pouls sees most frequently in autistic children in her practice are those for calcium, magnesium, and zinc. "Calcium is the nutrient that relaxes the nervous system, that prevents nervousness, irritability, anxiety, and hyperactivity," she says. "Magnesium, which most of them are equally deficient in, can prevent muscle tremor, spasm, and cramping. A lot of these children have nervous muscular twitches and reactions." As for zinc, Dr. Pouls cites it

About Electrolytes and Minerals

Electrolytes are substances (including acids, bases, and mineral salts such as potassium, magnesium, and calcium) that conduct an electrical charge. Electrolytes are vital to cellular regulation and control, the transmission of electrochemical impulses to nerves and muscles, and metabolism, among other functions.

Minerals are divided into two categories: bulk or major minerals, and trace or minor minerals. The bulk minerals are calcium, chloride, magnesium, phosphorus, potassium, sodium, and sulfur. The trace minerals are boron, chromium, copper, iodine, iron, manganese, molybdenum, selenium, silicon, vanadium, and zinc.

as one of the two most needed nutrients to support immune function, the other being vitamin C.

"When these children cannot absorb magnesium very well in the gastrointestinal tract, an excellent way for them to get it is by taking Epsom salt (magnesium sulfate) baths," states Dr. Pouls. She suggests adding half a cup to a cup of Epsom salt to a tub of water as warm as the child can handle it. The tub should be filled with enough water so that the child is immersed up to his neck. Have him soak for 15 to 20 minutes, says Dr. Pouls. You can do this daily, or as needed. "If a child is hyper, they say put the child in water," she notes. "This does even more. The magnesium in the Epsom salt goes in and relaxes their muscles. If the child is having a hyper, agitated, irritated day, have him take a bath. Make it fun, throw toys in the bath."

The bath is actually a multifold treatment: the body absorbs needed magnesium through the skin; it helps calm and relax a child; and Epsom salt gently detoxifies the body as well, drawing toxins out through the skin. With the liver and the lymphatic system, the skin is part of the body's detoxification system, helping to rid the body of toxins by excreting them through its pores.

Of vitamins autistic children tend to be deficient in, Dr.

Pouls typically finds a need for vitamin C, vitamin B_6, and folic acid (in the B vitamin family). As the B vitamins support brain, nerve, and immune function, correcting deficiencies in these nutrients has obvious import for children with autism. As noted above, vitamin C lends much-needed assistance to the immune system, which in these children is severely compromised.

Essential fatty acids are another important nutrient to consider. As detailed earlier, the 24-hour urinalysis reveals how well the body is breaking down carbohydrates, proteins, and fat. "If a child is not breaking down fats, it almost always means a deficiency in the essential fatty acids," states Dr. Pouls. Again, there is a blood test to evaluate which of the 36 essential fatty acids a child is deficient in, but Dr. Pouls has found that providing a balanced ratio of omega 3 and omega 6 is usually all that is needed. "Sometimes we focus just on the fish oils (omega-3 EFAs), for brain function. Many times, the children's diets are high in omega 6, and out of balance with or low in the omega 3s."

The EFA supplement that seems to do the most good, and Dr. Pouls's clinical experience is borne out by numerous studies, is cod liver oil. It is high in both EPA (eicosapentaenoic acid), a particularly beneficial omega 3, and vitamin A, another nutrient in which autistic children are often deficient. The vitamin A in cod liver oil is absorbable by people with a compromised digestive lining, as is frequently the case with this population.

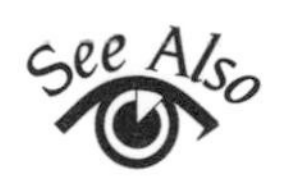

For more about nutritional deficiencies in autism, see chapter 2.

Dr. Pouls uses a good-tasting chewable form of cod liver oil, which is far easier to get children to take than the nasty spoonful of old. She advises consumer caution when it comes to fish oil products, given that fish is a major source of mercury and other heavy metals. "Those contaminants are particularly concentrated in the fish oil," she says. "You need to get a product that has a good certificate of analysis showing the heavy metal content." This should be available from the manufacturer. "The quality of the fish oil is crucial. You can't just assume that all fish oils are created equal. They are not."

For autistic children, Dr. Pouls also often recommends supplementation with DMG. Along with vitamin B_6 and magnesium, DMG is frequently cited as a beneficial supplement in the treatment of autism (see chapter 2).

Correcting deficiencies and other problems revealed by the preliminary tests (urinalysis and hair) is sufficient to rebalance most children in her practice, says Dr. Pouls. Giving the child the enzymes he needs, improving his digestion, and getting his nutrient (vitamin, mineral, amino acid, and essential fatty acid) levels back up gives him the building blocks required for brain and nerve cell function, and for healing. In a few cases, further testing is necessary, but Dr. Pouls waits to see the effects of initial treatment before she makes that determination. "If we did all the testing all at once, it would be very expensive, and might not be necessary."

Liver Support

Along with the digestion improvement and nutrient rebuilding program, Dr. Pouls starts the child on a liver support formula to help that organ start detoxifying and functioning more optimally. Children often feel a difference in three weeks on this combination protocol. As mentioned previously, this may be enough to reduce or reverse their autistic symptoms. Oral chelation, the therapy to rid the body of heavy metals, notably mercury and lead, may not be required.

Part of the reason for this may be that, even if the child previously had significant mercury or other heavy metal levels, improving digestion improves the ability of the body to chelate heavy metals on its own. This is because some amino acids—methionine and cysteine, for example—are bound with sulfur, a natural chelating agent. When the body is digesting protein optimally—that is, breaking down protein into its amino acid components—methionine and cysteine can serve as natural chelators. Thus, with restored digestion, the body has the ability to rid itself of some heavy metals.

In any case, Dr. Pouls keeps children on the program for at least two months before initiating chelation. "You don't want to do chelation, pulling out these heavy metals, if their liver function isn't optimal because then the liver won't move the heavy metals out quickly enough. That will produce side effects or an increase in symptoms," she states, adding that detoxification is a strain on the body, even though the chelation product is a natural one.

Liver support is necessary in the majority of cases. "I can see in the urinalysis of most of these children that they have compromised liver function due to severe colon toxicity due to poor digestion, which puts a huge stress on the liver," she explains. Or, as is true of a number of children with autism, they may have a defect in their liver's ability to process sulfur compounds. As sulfur is key to liver detoxification, this could lead to a

In Their Own Words

"After just three weeks [on Dr. Pouls' treatment program], Max's therapists, teacher, and neighbors were telling me that he was like a new kid. They could not get over how much more alert, calm, and cooperative he was.

"Over the next two months, we saw many more improvements, especially in his classroom involvement. He is so much more focused on his work, participates in circle time activities, is trying his best to sing in music, and has taken on a new interest in drawing and writing. Max totally surprised his occupational therapist and me by drawing people with all the details, emotions, etc. Three months ago, he would be doing well to draw just a circle. He is now choosing to do pencil and paper work.

"The very best part of all is that Max has just started to call his classmates by their names, and has added, 'You play with me?' He is getting a great response from the kids—they're playing with him! This means more to Max and me than everything else put together."

—Polly Kurtz, mother of Max, 8

buildup of toxins as detoxification is impaired. The children's liver function may also be compromised by the children not getting adequate nutrients or being given too many drugs. "Antibiotics, Ritalin, and all the other drugs given to autistic children add a chemical burden to their liver, have undesirable side effects, and don't address the underlying problems," says Dr. Pouls.

To strengthen and detoxify the liver, Dr. Pouls uses Liver Support System, a plant-based product she formulated for that purpose. The formula contains concentrates of an artichoke hybrid *(Cynara floridanum)* and sarsaparilla *(Smilax aristolochiaefolia)*. Artichoke has a long history of use in treating liver conditions, and sarsaparilla has long served as a blood purifier, antitoxin, and tonic.[132] Once the liver is restored to better, if not optimum functioning, oral chelation can be implemented if hair analysis shows that it is needed.

Getting the Mercury Out

Dr. Pouls is one of those who credit the exponential rise in autism since 1987 to the greater toxicity of our environment, including the increasing amounts of mercury to which we are exposed. "Mercury is everywhere," she attests. "We're getting it from our food, from our water, from dental fillings, through vaccinations. It's bioaccumulative, so there's even more of it now in our water, in our air, and in our bodies."

Bioaccumulative means that it doesn't break down in the environment or in the body. It remains in both, and each exposure adds to the accumulation. The body's natural chelators, such as the amino acids methionine and cysteine, can remove some, but if exposure is too high, they are unable to handle the problem. Unless you do an oral or intravenous chelation to remove the mercury, it remains in your tissues.

As discussed in chapter 2, vaccines have been a major source of mercury for children within their first two years of life, as most manufacturers, until recently, used thimerosal, a form of mercury, as a preservative in many vaccines. Dr. Pouls finds this unconscionable, given the fact that the neurotoxicity of mercury and all heavy metals has long been recognized. "Parents need to know that they have the right to request vaccines that don't contain heavy metal preservatives," she says.

In answer to those who refuse to acknowledge that childhood immunizations are a contributing factor in the rise of autism, arguing that if that were the case, then all children who are vaccinated would develop autism, Dr. Pouls points to individual susceptibility and an aggregation of contributing factors.

Number one, some children come into this world already carrying a mercury load, she notes. "While the fetus was maturing, the mother may have had a lot of mercury in her system, either due to eating a lot of fish that contains high amounts of mercury, especially canned tuna, or to her mercury amalgam dental fillings. The amount of mercury released from fillings depends on the acidity of the saliva [higher acidity is associated with mercury leaching], how many fillings are in the mouth, and whether one filling is abrading another." The mercury in the mother's body travels to the infant's body via the placental blood.

Number two, there has been poor quality control of the amount of mercury and other heavy metals put into vaccines, so amounts vary widely. "One child may get ten times the mercury in a vaccination compared to another child getting the same vaccination."

Number three, says Dr. Pouls, multiple vaccines are hard on children's bodies. "The child who gets a lot all at once has a greater chance of developing autism because of how that suppresses the immune system." If the child is already run down, with a cold, for example, getting the shots on top of that may be the final straw for the immune system. Unfortunately, many children received their shots when they were already sick with a cold or other mild ailment.

So the child may have a toxic accumulation already, be run down, and then get many vaccines all at once. The factor that may, in combination with some or all of these conditions, tip the scales toward autism relates to susceptibility, states Dr. Pouls.

"Some people are born with a stronger constitution, some people have a genetic weakness in a certain area. Even if it's not a disease state, it's a weak system. So, under stress, one person always get headaches, another person always gets colds, flu, and other respiratory ailments because the lungs are the weak area, other people get ulcers. We each have certain systems that are weaker than others. In the case of autistic children, they may have an extrasensitive nervous system, congenital enzyme deficiency, or a congenital defect in the liver's ability to detoxify, which makes them more susceptible to developing autism."

Successful treatment of autism, as with any disorder, requires removing the contributing factors. The program of improving digestion, making sure the child is getting the nutrient building blocks she needs for a strong and healthy body, removing stress on and strengthening the immune system, and restoring the liver in being able to do its work of ridding the body of toxins goes a long way toward accomplishing that. As noted previously, it may be sufficient to ameliorate autistic symptoms.

If this is not the case and the child's hair analysis shows a heavy metal load (she never does chelation without running a hair analysis to determine the need for it), Dr. Pouls will implement oral chelation. Again, she will not do so until the child's body is strong enough to handle the extra stress of detoxification.

Chelation is often an intravenous (IV) therapy. The chelating agent, typically DMPS (2,3-dimercaptopropane-1-sulfonate) for mercury, is delivered as an infusion, meaning an IV drip, over several hours. Dr. Pouls formulated a plant-based oral chelation product because DMPS and other IV chelating agents are "hard on the body, especially for a young child whose kidneys and liver detoxification pathways are very sensitive. I find that I get less symptoms or side affects using natural plant-based chelators." In addition, oral chelation is far less expensive, invasive, and time-consuming than IV chelation. It doesn't involve needles, which many children are afraid of, and can be done at home in the time it takes to swallow a capsule morning and night.

Dr. Pouls' Oral Chelation can be ordered through her or the manufacturer. For Dr. Pouls' contact information, see appendix B. The manufacturer has two ordering branches: for laypeople, Extreme Health (www.extremehealthusa.com) at 800-800-1285 or 925-855-1262; and for health-care practitioners, Extended Health (www.extendedhealth.com) at 800-300-6712 or 925-855-1263.

Dr. Pouls has used her oral chelation formula safely and successfully with children as young as three years old. "I haven't worked with children under three who have been diagnosed with autism," she says. "Most children don't get a diagnosis until around then."

Among the chelating and/or binding agents in Dr. Pouls' Oral Chelation formula are chlorella, cilantro, garlic, sodium alginate, clay, alpha-lipoic acid, vitamin C, selenium, zinc, and the amino acids L-cysteine, L-lysine, and L-methionine. As chelation draws minerals as well as heavy metals out of the body, the chelation program includes a companion formula that replenishes minerals, and also contains 30 different antioxidants, kidney and liver support substances, and specific enzymes to ensure the utilization of all the nutrients in the formula.

Max and Mercury

Max had been exhibiting autistic-like behaviors since he was less than a year old. At one point, a pediatric center diagnosed him with dyspraxia, the inability to coordinate motor functions, including speech. According to the parameters of the Autism Research Institute in San Diego, California, he placed in the category of severe autism, reports his mother, Polly Kurtz.

Max was not always this way, she says. Although she can't correlate it precisely, she thinks it was after one of his early vaccinations that he became docile (he had the hepatitis B vaccine at birth and the usual schedule of immunizations thereafter). "He just slipped off and got really quiet." This was sometime between four and nine months old, because she remembers how he used to act around that time, and he was a different baby. "I would take him to the grocery store and he would try to get people's attention with his eyes, blink at them and grin at them until they would say, 'Oh you're so cute.' Making eye contact with them and playing with them like that stopped. He turned into a baby that would just sit there and didn't want to interact, didn't want to reach for things."

He also got sick a lot, had a cold ten times a year and a chronically runny nose. When he was almost two, he began to say a few words, but he lost those and from then on didn't speak.

At seven, when Max started on Dr. Pouls' nutritional program, his major problems were lack of speech, difficulty focusing in school, and aggressive behavior. His aggression toward others in the classroom, which included grabbing, pushing, kicking, biting, and throwing sand and other objects, made it unsafe for him to be at school.

There was a big improvement after just three weeks on the program, says Polly, noting that it wasn't just she who saw the change. "Everyone around him could not believe the difference in him." The main difference was that he was more calm and did not seem to get overstimulated by his environment, as he did previously. "He was calm enough to go into the classroom, sit down in a chair, and participate, pay attention for the most part in a circle time, which had been a really trying thing for him before." His motor function also improved, such that he began to cut and color, activities he wouldn't engage in prior to the treatment.

In the first two to three months on the program, Polly reports that "his speech and occupational therapists were blown away because he started cooperating with them, doing the things they had been asking him to do for two years." He started being more verbal about what he wanted instead of acting out. After six to seven months, his speech had increased to the point that he was saying phrases. Polly estimates that in that first six months on the program, Max progressed two years in his development, although he still exhibited some aggressive behavior.

Max's Hair Analyses

The following are Max's levels of heavy metals as revealed by two hair analyses, one before he started oral chelation and one after only six months of chelation. Dr. Pouls notes that the results of the second test were achieved with sporadic dosing. With more consistent adherence to the oral chelation program, she would expect these surprisingly good results to be even better.

Before Chelation

Mercury: 4.95 (normal = 0-1)
Aluminum: 13.6 (normal = 0-8)
Lead: 0.53 (normal = 0-0.5)

After Six Months of Chelation

Mercury: 3.03
Aluminum: 4.8
Lead: 0.31

When Max had been on the program for a year, Dr. Pouls tested him for heavy metals. The hair analysis revealed that Max's level of mercury was "off the scale" at 4.95 (normal is 0-1), according to Dr. Pouls. The test also showed high aluminum (13.6; normal is 0-8) and slightly elevated lead (0.53; normal is 0-0.5). While that level of lead might not be problematic on its own, Dr. Pouls notes, it contributed to the cumulative load of neurotoxic heavy metals in Max's case. In addition, as stated in Abra's story, research has clearly linked elevated lead levels with aggressive tendencies, which might explain some of Max's aggression. As to the sources of the heavy metal exposure, it is only possible to speculate: the mercury may have come from the vaccines or another typical source; and the lead may have been from the water pipes in the 150-year-old house the Kurtz family lived in when Max was a baby.

Despite the already significant improvements, Polly cites the biggest change in Max as occurring after chelation. His aggressive behavior completely disappeared, even in the face of new people and situations, which used to set him off. "Now I can take him anywhere. And he's listening to me; I don't have to hold onto him when I get out of the car in a parking lot. He's talking, speaking sentences. And he plays jokes on you. His ability to think has improved, to carry out a thought, and to think about what's going to happen if I do this." Now eight, Max is at about the kindergarten/first grade level and behaves like any six-year-old boy, she says.

Polly believes that metals are a core issue in autism and that all autistic children need to be tested. "I tell everyone that all the therapies that Max has been through put together haven't made such a difference as the chelation and the nutritional therapy." As a measure in the change in Max, Polly announces that he "just got an award in front of the whole school last week for 'The Best Listener.'"

A Word to Parents

In addition to targeted therapeutic nutrition and heavy metal detoxification, Dr. Pouls emphasizes a few lifestyle issues that are of concern for children with autistic symptoms. "Some kind of physical exercise is really crucial, any kind of outings, like walking in the park," she states. "The parents often don't know what to do, so they give the children TV to baby-sit them." She understands the difficulty of coping with children who have autism, but a television baby-sitter is not an ongoing solution. Reading to them, playing with them, and developing motor skills are very important. At the same time, so is outside assistance, says Dr. Pouls, citing the existence of many excellent programs to help the parents give their children what they need.

"I do not have all the pieces of the puzzle, but I believe that nutrition and what testing we have available now can help so much and take the children so far that the children are then able to become involved in other learning programs—mental, emotional, and physical activities that they couldn't even consider entering into before," she says. "Other doors open because they now have the capacity to begin."

5 NAET: *Allergy-Related Autism*

As stated previously, whether the allergies frequently associated with autism are a contributing factor or a consequence of the underlying conditions present in autism is a subject of debate, but allergy expert Dr. Devi S. Nambudripad, M.D., D.C., L.Ac., Ph.D., of Buena Park, California, has found that symptoms of autism can be reversed or reduced by eliminating allergies in many cases. In the early 1980s, Dr. Devi, as she is widely known, developed a method of eliminating allergies—NAET (Nambudripad's Allergy Elimination Techniques)—which is now practiced worldwide by over 5,000 health-care practitioners.

Dr. Devi S. Nambudripad *has found that symptoms of autism can be reversed or reduced by eliminating allergies in many cases.* Eliminating *allergic reactions lifts a large burden from the immune system;* reduces toxic *substances in the body and therefore also lifts a burden from the liver and other parts of the detoxification system; and improves digestion.*

In *Say Good-Bye to Allergy-Related Autism,* Dr. Devi points out the significant overlap between the symptoms of allergies and those of autism (see sidebar). Although she recognizes the existence of autism as a distinct disorder, she believes that many children who receive the diagnosis are actually only suffering from allergies.

Symptoms of Allergies

The following are some of the many common symptoms of allergies. These symptoms and/or conditions are also typical of or have been observed in autistic children.

- anxiety
- attention deficit
- *Candida*/yeast overgrowth
- craving for carbohydrates/chocolate
- distractibility
- dyslexia
- ear infections
- eating disorders
- eczema
- frequent colds, bronchial infections, and other infections
- hyperactivity
- impulsivity
- indigestion
- insomnia
- irritable bowel syndrome
- leaky gut syndrome
- mood swings
- nervous stomach
- obsessive-compulsive disorder
- parasitic infestation
- phobias
- poor appetite
- poor memory
- restless leg syndrome
- sinusitis
- toxicity (reactivity/sensitivity) to mercury and other heavy metals

Other symptoms of allergies that are not necessarily associated with autism, but may be present include: asthma, chronic fatigue, colitis, fibromyalgia, flatulence, general itching, headaches, hives, hypoglycemia, and night sweats.[133]

Her clinical experience has borne this out; in many of the cases she has treated, the symptoms on which the diagnosis of autism was based disappeared after the allergies were eliminated.

For those children whose autism involves other factors in addition to allergies, eliminating their allergies is still a useful course. Doing so can alleviate symptoms both directly and indirectly: directly, by removing the source of allergy-related symptoms; and indirectly, by easing other problems that may be exacerbating or producing symptoms. Eliminating allergic reactions lifts a large burden from the immune system; reduces toxic substances in the body and therefore also lifts a burden from the liver and other parts of the detoxification system; and improves digestion. The latter is essential in reversing intestinal disorders associated with autism and in increasing nutrient absorption and assimilation, which in turn builds up all body systems and improves overall health.

While more parents of autistic children have become aware that there may be a link between allergies and their child's autistic symptoms, many still do not know that there is an alternative to the rigors of avoidance diets. Such diets are hard on both parent and child as they entail keeping children away from what are often not only their favorite foods, but also some of the only foods they will eat. By eliminating allergies, NAET obviates the need for these difficult food restrictions.

The NAET method both identifies and eliminates allergies. It uses kinesiology's muscle response testing (MRT) to identify allergies. Chiropractic and acupuncture techniques are then implemented to remove the energy blockages in the body that underlie allergies, and to reprogram the brain and nervous system not to respond allergically to previously problem substances. As a noninvasive and painless testing and therapeutic method, NAET works well with children.

Like many revolutionary inventions, NAET began with an accidental discovery. Dr. Devi, who had long been allergic to nearly everything, one day ate some carrot while she was cooking the two foods she could safely eat—white rice and broccoli. Within moments of eating the carrot, she "felt like [she] was going to pass out."[134]

She used muscle response testing to check for an allergy to carrots and was not surprised that she tested highly allergic.

A student of acupuncture at the time, she gave herself an acupuncture treatment, with the help of her husband, to keep from going into shock. She fell asleep with the needles still inserted in specific acupuncture points, and when she woke almost an hour later, she no longer felt sick and tired. In her hand were pieces of the carrot she had been eating. When she repeated the MRT, she no longer tested allergic to carrots. To check the validity of this result, she ate some carrot—no reaction.[135]

Dr. Devi then ate bits of other foods to which she knew she was allergic and her reactions were as they had been—she was still allergic. "[S]o I knew my assumption was correct. My allergy to carrot was gone because of my contact with the carrot while undergoing acupuncture. My energy and the carrot's energy were repelling prior to the acupuncture treatment. After the treatment, their energies became similar—no more repulsion!"[136]

Dr. Devi then tried this technique, which she later named NAET, on other foods to which she was allergic. The same thing happened—the allergies disappeared. After many years of living with pervasive allergies, she was able to systematically eliminate them and restore her health.

How NAET Works

Dr. Devi based NAET on the medical model of acupuncture, in which disease is diagnosed and treated as an energy imbalance in one or more of the body's meridians, or energy pathways. These meridians—there are 12 major ones—carry the body's vital energy, or *qi* (*chi*), to organs and throughout the system. Acupuncturists rebalance a meridian's energy by treating acupoints, the points on the body's surface that correspond to that meridian. Via the painless insertion of needles or the application of pressure, the acupuncturist can remove energy blockages, get stagnant energy moving, or calm an overactive energy meridian.

According to Dr. Devi, who is a licensed acupuncturist, allergies are "energy incompatibilities" that create energy blockages in the body. That is, the body's energy field regards the energy field of a substance—eaten, inhaled, or otherwise contacted—as incompatible with its own, and its presence disturbs the flow of energy along the body's meridians. One, several, or even all of the meridians may be affected. The central nervous system records the energy disturbance and is then programmed to regard the substance as toxic. NAET uses chiropractic and acupuncture techniques to restore the smooth flow of energy along the meridians and reprogram the central nervous system to no longer regard the substance as incompatible energetically.

The energy disturbance created by an allergy is the key to muscle response testing. To be tested for a potential allergen (something that causes an allergic reaction), you hold a vial containing the substance in one hand. You hold your other arm straight out in front of you, and attempt to keep it there while the person testing pushes down on it slightly. Normally, you can easily hold your arm in place, but when you are allergic to the substance in the vial, your muscle response is weakened by the energy disturbance the allergy causes. A weakened response in testing indicates a possible allergy.

In Their Own Words

"At the age of three my son was classified as having PDD/Autism. After the shock wore off I decided to stop fighting with the pediatrician, and started listening to my family and friends to go the alternative way . . . [I got trained in NAET] so I could treat my children. My children, now 7 and 5, are no longer labeled autistic and attend regular schools. NAET is the answer to so many parents' prayers. Your child doesn't have to live a casein, gluten, and chemical free life! . . . Now I have started treating my autistic patients with NAET. I am amazed in a short period of time how NAET has transformed many children's lives in my practice."[137]

—Maribeth Mydlowski, D.C.,
NAET practitioner

Those who have not experienced this test often find it difficult to believe that it can tell you anything, much less identify allergies. Upon undergoing the test, however, most people are amazed to discover that their arm seems to have a life, or mind, of its own. One moment, while holding one test substance, they see their arm drop slightly, and the next, with a different test vial, the arm holds steady. The person being tested usually does not know what's in the vial, so that does not influence the outcome.

For the treatment phase, the person holds the vial of the offending substance while the NAET practitioner uses slight pressure, needles, or a chiropractic tool to treat the appropriate points to clear the affected meridian(s). Keeping the vial in your energy field during this process reprograms the brain and nervous system to regard the substance as innocuous. In general, it is then necessary to avoid ingesting or otherwise having contact with the substance for 25 hours after treatment.

Dr. Devi explains the reason for this time period: "An energy molecule takes 24 hours to travel through the body completing its circulation through all 12 major meridians, their branches, and subbranches. It takes two hours to travel through one meridian. . . . When the allergy is treated through NAET, the patient has to wait 24 hours to let the energy molecule carrying the new information pass through the complete cycle of the journey."[138] To be safe, one hour is added to the 24-hour cycle. If the person eats the allergenic food or has contact with an allergenic substance before the cycle is complete, the clearing treatment will likely have to be repeated and the food or other substance will need to be avoided for another 25 hours.

In her clinical practice, Dr. Devi has found that in cases of autism the avoidance period needs to be longer than usual. "In some children I have observed that it is necessary to avoid the treated food allergen for 30 hours," notes Dr. Devi. "This may be due to the fact that autistic children have extremely fatigued and diminished brain function."[139]

Dr. Devi and other NAET practitioners have seen remarkable improvements result from clearing autistic children of allergies. As stated earlier, even if the child's autism is not allergy related, clearing the allergies can only be an aid to a beleaguered body.

The Nambudripad Allergy Research Foundation in Buena Park, California, conducted a study of 14 children with autism spectrum disorder (ASD). None of the children were talking and all avoided eye contact. Following NAET treatment, 13 of the children began talking and 12 initiated eye contact. The number of twice-weekly treatment sessions ranged from 3 to 25, with 5 to 10 sessions producing these results in the greatest number of children.[140]

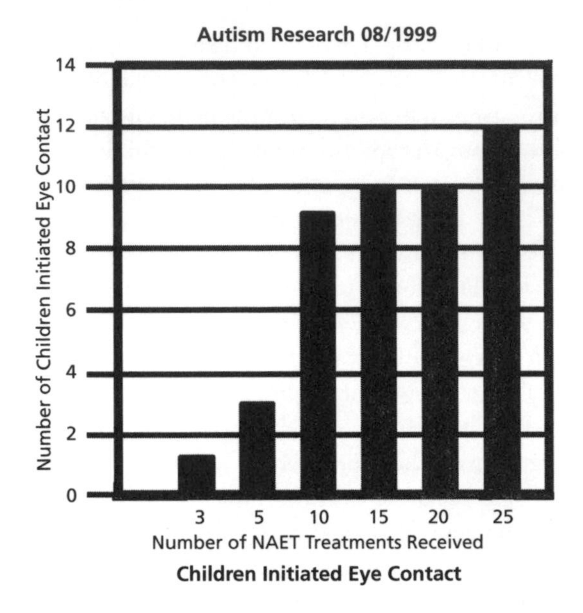

Children Initiated Eye Contact

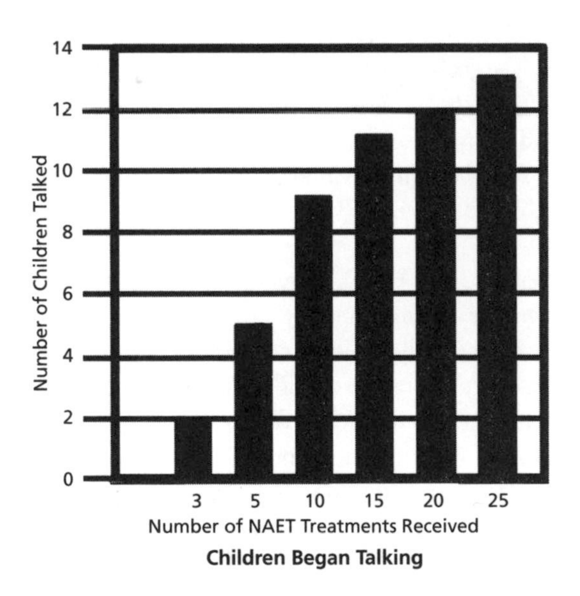

Children Began Talking

Source: reprinted with permission of Devi S. Nambudripad, from *Say Goodbye to Allergy-Related Autism*, Buena Park, CA: Delta Publishing, 1999: 30-31.

Common Allergens

In autism, multiple NAET treatments are usually necessary, as multiple allergies are typical. "Some autistic children and adults with mild to moderate symptoms may show marked improvements after they complete just five basic groups of allergens," states Dr. Devi.[141] These five are: egg mix (egg white, egg yolk, chicken, and the antibiotic tetracycline); calcium mix (breast milk, cow's milk, goat's milk, milk albumin, casein, lactic acid, calcium, and coumarin, a phenolic or natural component found in milk); vitamin C (fruits, vegetables, vinegar, citrus, and berry); B-complex vitamins (seventeen vitamins in the B family); and sugar mix (cane, corn, maple, grape, rice, brown, and beet sugars, plus molasses, honey, fructose, dextrose, glucose, and maltose). You may wonder why tetracycline is included in the egg mix. The answer is that chickens are routinely fed this antibiotic to keep infections that might kill them from doing so and also to prevent the spread of infection from chicken to chicken. Thus, tetracycline is a component of commercial chicken products.

Dr. Devi recommends more extensive clearing in the majority of cases, however. "Most autistic children and adults can get their symptoms under control when they complete the NAET basic thirty to forty-five groups of allergens successfully," she states.[142] "Successfully" means that after treatment the body tests "clear" of allergic reaction to the substance.

Not surprisingly, this larger collection of allergens includes magnesium, grain mix (including gluten), yeast mix (including acidophilus), essential fatty acid oils, amino acids, DMG, artificial sweeteners, food additives, and food coloring. In one way or another, all of these substances have implications for autism.

Deficiencies in magnesium, essential fatty acids, and amino acids are common among autistic children, while the results of DMG supplementation indicate the need for it. If a person is allergic to a nutrient, the body cannot absorb it and thus becomes deficient in it. An allergy to these nutrients might explain the deficiencies. An allergy to gluten (a grain protein), found in many children with autism, could also contribute to an amino acid deficiency, as the body cannot properly digest this food and therefore cannot assimilate the amino acids it contains.

It is worthwhile to note at this point that people can develop allergies to anything, even to nutrients that are natural to and required by the body. Says Dr. Devi, "Any substance under the sun, including sunlight itself, can cause an allergic reaction in any individual."[143]

Dr. Devi has seen a clear link between autistic symptoms and allergies to childhood immunizations—not only in her patients, but also in her own son. With elimination of the allergy to the problematic vaccine, the symptoms disappear.

With *Candida* overgrowth also a common problem in autistic children, it may not be surprising that they frequently test allergic to the yeast mix, which contains acidophilus. Acidophilus is the beneficial bacteria normally present in the intestines that help keep *Candida,* a yeast-like fungus, in check. With the body unable to utilize acidophilus, due to an allergy to it, *Candida* naturally flourishes.

The presence of artificial sweeteners, food additives, and food coloring in the NAET basic 30 to 45 groups of allergens is also not surprising. The autistic symptoms of many children have improved with the removal of these substances from the diet. Other schools of thought may regard the reason as being that these synthetic substances are neurotoxic to these individuals. Many NAET practitioners would agree, but say further that the neurotoxicity stems from the fact that the individuals are allergic to the substances. Once cleared of the allergy, in most cases, the child can eat foods containing these additives without suffering the negative effects. The same is true of gluten and casein (in the calcium mix), which is great news for parents who have struggled with the gluten-free and casein-free diet for their child.

In the basic groups of allergens recommended for testing in the case of autism are also immunizations and vaccinations, a mix containing MMR, DPT, polio, and hepatitis B, among others.

In Their Own Words

"[M]y youngest son was diagnosed with autism three weeks before his third birthday. . . . John seemed to develop normally from birth but started to regress in his second year. We knew something was wrong but thought he might have a hearing problem of some sort because he had no speech, would not respond when we called him, and had many temper tantrums.

"For two years [my husband and I] went all over the country seeing doctors we thought might have some answers. We dedicated ourselves to months of exhausting detoxification programs, doing chelation therapy and allergy shots. I'm not saying these therapies are not good, but they can be expensive, difficult to do, and John did not show the slightest bit of improvement from them.

"Next we tried a gluten-free diet, a sugar-free diet, and avoidance of all known allergens. He did show a little improvement with these, but they are tough on both parents and children to adhere to, plus autistic children are allergic to so much, foods and environmentally, it's impossible to keep them away from everything.

"We began NAET treatments . . . After clearing the first five items, John picked up some blocks with numbers on them; he had never shown any interest in these blocks in the past. As my husband and I sat in the living room observing him, John lined the numbers up in the correct order on a window ledge and said each number out loud. We had never heard him talking in his little voice before. What a joy this brought us. . . . After John cleared for wheat and gluten he could eat wheat without any problems. Candida *was a big problem for John and once he was cleared of sugar and yeast he no longer had to be on an anti-*Candida *diet and there have been no signs of* Candida.

"He can say his ABCs and count to thirty. . . . He is much calmer and able to sit for an hour and a half straight, which makes it easier for him to learn. His eye contact is much improved along with his eating habits. Instead of looking at my son with sorrow as I did in the past, I can look at him with hope for the future."[144]

—John's mother (the boy's name has been changed)

The vaccines are also tested and treated individually in many instances. (Mercury, lead, and other metals that are used as preservatives in vaccines are tested in the mineral mix, which is also one of the basic groups.) In chapter 7, you will learn how homeopathic nosodes can be used to clear the adverse reactions of a vaccine from the body. Dr. Devi uses NAET to do the same, regarding the toxic reaction of the child to the vaccine as an allergic response. That response can be eliminated by clearing the allergy, she notes.

Dr. Devi has seen a clear link between autistic symptoms and allergies to childhood immunizations—not only in her patients, but also in her own son. With elimination of the allergy to the problematic vaccine, the symptoms disappear. In many cases, the MMR vaccine is the culprit, but in her son's case, DPT was the problem.

Roy and the DPT Vaccine

Dr. Devi's son Roy began walking and talking early—at 7 and 13 months, respectively.*

"By the time he was 15 months he knew his alphabet fluently and he could count to one hundred clearly," recalls Dr. Devi. At 18 months, like most children in the United States, he was given his booster shot of DPT. (This was before Dr. Devi knew of the potential deleterious effects of vaccines.) For two days afterward, he ran a 100-degree fever. Two weeks after the shot, he developed flu-like symptoms, including a fever of 103 to 104, that lasted for a month. Dr. Devi, who already knew MRT, tested Roy for the antibiotics the doctor prescribed. Since Roy tested allergic, she didn't give them to him, but treated the flu and fever with Chinese herbal medicine and Tylenol (after testing him for both to make sure he wasn't allergic).

---

*This case study adapted, by permission of Devi S. Nambudripad, D.C., L.Ac., R.N., Ph.D., from *Say Goodbye to Allergy-Related Autism*, by Devi S. Nambudripad (Buena Park, California: Delta Publishing, 1999): 221-4.

Roy emerged from his "flu" a changed child, according to Dr. Devi: "He became very hyper, his vocabulary went down instead of getting better. He did not have the attention span [he had] before. He began getting destructive. . . . He threw his toys all over and it was difficult to make him put them back in place. . . . He forgot his alphabet and numbers." He also developed a chronically runny nose, hives, knee and other joint pain, leg cramps, severe insomnia, and temper tantrums.

Roy had many allergies and Dr. Devi treated him with NAET from the time he was four until he was six, when he "became almost normal." She had to teach him his alphabet and numbers again. Most of his symptoms went away after she cleared him for an allergy to DPT, but residual symptoms remained. These were not resolved until she tested him on the separate components of the DPT shot. Pertussis turned out to be the source of his lingering health problems. Clearing him for that, as well as for the brain, hypothalamus, nerves, lung tissue, and the neurotransmitter serotonin, got rid of his last symptoms.

Yes, the body can develop a reactivity to its own tissue and brain chemicals. In Roy's case, the pertussis was behind this. "The toxin produced by pertussis affected his stomach, spleen, and liver meridians and brain. The energy blockages in these meridians and associated organs caused his health disorders . . . until the allergy to the pertussis vaccine was eliminated."

As an aside, Dr. Devi notes that allergic reactions tend to affect certain organs or meridians in individuals, depending on where their weak or vulnerable areas are. The organ most affected is known as the "target organ." The weakness can be genetic in nature or created by environmental factors such as toxic exposure or lack of adequate nutrition. The DPT and MMR vaccines will "attack" the weak area, or you could say that area is thrown out of balance or overloaded with the toxins of the vaccines.

For example, "Roy had a weak stomach and spleen meridian from the time he was born," explains Dr. Devi. This meant that the energy flow on these meridians was not optimal, and thus the organs fed by the meridians were compromised to some degree. "He used to spit up his formula after each meal." Later, after learning kinesiology and muscle testing, she tested Roy and discovered that he was allergic to the food he was eating. As for the weakness in his liver, it was probably genetic, she says, inherited from his grandfather who died of liver cancer.

Dr. Devi warns parents that it is important to know that the incubation period of viruses varies. This is why, when your child gets a three-in-one vaccination, you may see some symptoms right away and others beginning weeks later. Due to the delay, some people fail to make the connection between the later symptoms and the immunizations. In Roy's case, his symptoms occurred the way they did, she explains, because the incubation period for diphtheria is only two to six days, while that of pertussis is seven to sixteen days.

In her practice, most of the parents of the autistic children she has seen recall their symptoms beginning around the ages of 15 to 18 months, after a "flu." Dr. Devi suggests that this "flu" may have been the reaction to DPT or MMR vaccinations. The children were then treated with antibiotics. "These children may have been allergic to antibiotics," states Dr. Devi. "[T]he allergic reaction from the vaccination combined with the allergic reaction from the antibiotics together attacked the brain—the target organ; and the result was autism." She notes that if she had given Roy the prescribed antibiotics, he, too, may have become autistic.[145]

Simon: Treatment at Nine Years Old

As with other therapeutic interventions, the earlier NAET can be implemented in a case of autism the better. Results can be achieved with older children, however, as the case of Simon illustrates.[†] Simon, age nine, had been diagnosed with autism spec-

---

[†]This case study adapted, by permission of Devi S. Nambudripad, D.C., L.Ac., R.N., Ph.D., from *Say Goodbye to Allergy-Related Autism,* by Devi S. Nambudripad (Buena Park, California: Delta Publishing, 1999): 237-44.

trum disorder when he was four years old. Categorized as high functional, he exhibited all the classic behaviors of autism and suffered occasional seizures. When Dr. Devi evaluated him, she noted the following:

"[H]e avoided eye contact, played alone, showed no awareness of people, resisted physical touch by anyone including his mother, lacked appropriate social or emotional responses, lacked communication skills, was unable to talk, made unusual sounds, had extreme need for sameness, was attached to an old baby blanket, was preoccupied with twirling and pulling his hair or chewing the sleeve of his long-sleeve shirt, . . . flapped his hand over the left side of his face repeatedly, showed distress and cried every now and then without any reason, and wet his pants periodically."

Simon's parents reported that he also had suffered from insomnia, eczema, itchiness, canker sores, and a slight cough for the previous six months, among other symptoms, and that he was uncooperative in learning or doing schoolwork. In addition, they had observed that his seizures seemed to be triggered by high consumption of refined sugar, and that quite a few foods made his autistic symptoms much worse. The problem foods comprised a long list, including dairy products, eggs, wheat, oats, corn, brown rice, beans, chocolate, fruits, fish, barbecued beef, hot dogs, pork, chicken, nuts, raisins, potatoes, and tomatoes, among others. Ice cubes and his prescription medication also exacerbated his symptoms.

Muscle response testing indicated allergies in twenty groups of basic allergens. On his first visit, he was treated for egg mix. His mother later reported that he stopped coughing within hours of this treatment. The next visit, he was treated for calcium mix. After that, his canker sores healed completely. Then he was cleared for vitamin C mix.

Dr. Devi details the change in him:

"On the following visit, he appeared restless and refused to sit in the chair to wait his turn. Instead, he rushed into my office. My quick impulse was [to ask] 'How are you, Simon?'

"'How are you Simon?' He repeated my question.

"'Ah! Simon, you are speaking!' I exclaimed.

"He snorted back 'Ah! Simon, you are speaking!'

"Then his mother walked in and stood behind him with a beaming smile . . . He repeated every word his mother said for the next few minutes. He had a smile on his face all along. His mother said he was chirping away nonstop after the treatment for vitamin C. . . . He repeated everyone's conversation throughout the week. She was so relieved to hear him speak, even though his speech didn't make any sense. All these years, she never knew that he could say even one word. . . . 'He did not even appear that he was listening,' she said. 'How could he have learned all these words and sentences?'"

After clearing more of his many allergies, Simon's eczema and itchiness subsided. On one visit, he ran into Dr. Devi's office, hugged her, looked into her eyes, and said, "I love you, Dr. Devi." In addition to all of the basic allergens, Simon needed to be treated for a wide range of others, including neurotransmitters, tap water, his past and present medications, pesticides, fabrics, and childhood immunizations (MMR, DPT, and polio). After being cleared for the latter, his seizures stopped. It took many NAET treatments to clear Simon of all his allergies, but today he is a healthy teenager and attends regular school.[146]

6 Biochemical Therapy and a Landmark Discovery

Biochemical researcher William J. Walsh, Ph.D., may well have discovered the cause of autism or, at the very least, a fundamental cause of autism. Preliminary findings strongly suggest that this is so, but Dr. Walsh is awaiting the results of his genetic research project currently under way before he is willing to state it definitively.

Biochemical researcher William J. Walsh, Ph.D., *may well have discovered the cause of autism or, at the very least, a fundamental cause of autism.* This *factor is a deficiency in or malfunction of metallothionein, a vital protein involved in many functions of the body.*

The factor Dr. Walsh isolated not only provides an answer as to why some children develop autism while others, exposed to the same elements, do not, it also explains the presence of all of the other conditions associated with autism: immune impairment, reactivity to immunizations and their heavy metal preservatives, allergies, fungal overgrowth, mineral deficiencies such as low zinc, high levels of heavy metals, and impaired nerve development, which can result in incomplete development of the brain and gastrointestinal system.

This factor is a deficiency in or malfunction of metallothionein, a vital protein involved in many functions of the body, including immunity, brain and gastrointestinal tract maturation, and the regulation of metals (both minerals and heavy metals such as mercury). A deficiency in or inability to utilize this substance has obvious consequences in the case of the first two functions: weakened immunity; an impaired nervous system; mental difficulties; and digestive problems as indicated by fungal overgrowth, nutritional deficiencies, and the development of allergies.

In terms of metal regulation, without metallothionein, the body cannot maintain proper mineral levels in the blood nor process toxic heavy metals such as mercury. The result is skewed mineral ratios (as in the high copper/low zinc ratio present in many autistic children) and an accumulation of mercury, lead, and other damaging heavy metals to which the child is exposed.

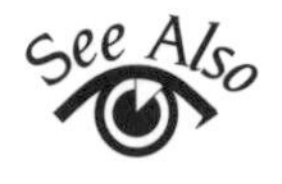

For more about the relationship between digestion and allergies, see chapters 4 and 5.

This amazing discovery arose from analysis of perhaps the world's largest and best database of the biochemistry of autistic people. The database consists of the results of blood and urine tests of 503 people who strictly fit into one of three diagnostic categories of autism: classic (Kanner) autism, pervasive development disorder (PDD), and Asperger's syndrome. This data was not gathered in a study, but amassed as an integral part of medical treatment at the Health Research Institute and Pfeiffer Treatment Center (HRIPTC) in Naperville, Illinois, a not-for-profit research and outpatient facility near Chicago. HRI is the research wing and PTC the treatment wing.

Designed as a collaboration between biochemists and medical doctors, the organization specializes in biochemical treatment of mental, emotional, and behavioral disorders. Since its founding in 1989, it has treated more than fifteen thousand people with autism, bipolar disorder, depression and anxiety disorders, schizophrenia, attention deficit disorder, hyperactivity, and other behavioral, emotional, and learning problems.

Dr. Walsh, chief scientist at HRIPTC, is the heir-apparent of the late Carl Pfeiffer, M.D., Ph.D., a pioneer in the biochemical treatment of illness, and of schizophrenia in particular. Before he died, Dr. Pfeiffer asked Dr. Walsh to establish the center to carry on the important work in which they had both been engaged for decades.

"What I've been doing for the last 25 or 30 years," explains Dr. Walsh, "is trying to develop chemical classifications for conditions such as behavior disorders, depression, schizophrenia, and autism because every one of these terms is an umbrella term or a garbage term that encompasses different categories." The chemistry underlying the diagnosis is not only the key to individual treatment, but if biochemical commonalities could be found among individuals in each category, this could also potentially point the way to the cause of the disorder, with attendant prevention and even cure.

What Is Biochemical Therapy?

Biochemical therapy is the supplemental use of substances that naturally occur in the body (for example, vitamins, minerals, amino acids, and enzymes) to rebalance an individual's disturbed biochemistry. The therapy operates on the tenet of biochemical individuality, which holds that every individual's biochemistry is unique and treatment must identify and address the unique condition. Treatment also considers the effects of environmental and food supply toxins, and includes natural detoxification protocols as needed.

The Metallothionein Key

In pursuit of the chemistry behind autism, in the summer of 2000, Dr. Walsh gave a staff of interns a voluminous project: (1) computerize the center's massive records; (2) pull out the records of those who fit one of the three defined autism categories (classic autism, PDD, and Asperger's); and (3) run statistical analyses on test results to see if they could identify any shared chemical markers among the 120 to 140 measures in each patient's test.

The second step left a database of 503 out of more than 700 people, mostly children, who had come to the Pfeiffer Treatment Center (PTC) with the label of autistic. The results of the third step were startling: all but 4 of the 503 people with autism showed clear evidence of a metallothionein dysfunction, and 85 percent had sky-high copper in relation to low zinc levels in their blood. Further, there was no chemical difference among the three autistic categories.

These results indicated that "all three groups had an absolutely severe metal metabolism problem, far beyond anything we've ever seen," observes Dr. Walsh. A metal metabolism problem, as reflected by a skewed ratio of copper to zinc, means the body is unable to control the mineral levels in the bloodstream. Normally, the body can maintain homeostasis (the proper ratio) of copper and zinc in the blood, regardless of diet or other factors, because this ratio is so crucial to many functions. This mechanism of homeostasis relies upon metallothionein; thus, an inability to maintain homeostasis indicates a metallothionein problem.

"We could explain everything from this one protein." The early abstract Dr. Walsh wrote on his findings concluded with the line: "These data suggest that an inborn error of metallothionein functioning may be a fundamental cause of autism."

Dr. Walsh concluded, after studying the results of the statistical analysis and going back through the records, chart by chart, "that there were only 4 out of the 503 that didn't have evidence of metallothionein dysfunction. The first thought we had, of course, was could this be the cause of autism? Or *a* cause of autism, or maybe a primary factor required for autism? We've been studying this now for a year and I believe the answer is 'yes.'"

After the initial results, Dr. Walsh and his colleagues then asked, "If you assume that somebody has a genetic metallothionein abnormality, what would you expect?" To answer this question, they looked at all the functions of metallothionein, beyond regulating copper and zinc, and what would happen if that vital

Correlation of Metallothionein Defect with Autism Symptoms/Conditions

The column on the left lists the functions in the body in which metallothionein is necessary. The column on the right lists the symptoms and/or conditions associated with autism, grouped according to their connection with a disturbance in the function on the left. For example, a problem in the operation of the immune system can result in chronic/frequent colds, flu, and other infection.

Metallothionein Functions	**Autism Symptoms/Conditions**
Immune function	weakened immunity chronic/frequent colds, flu, ear, and other infections allergies/environmental sensitivity fungal overgrowth autoimmune problems reactivity/sensitivity to vaccines
Brain maturation/nerve cell development	impaired nervous system speech deficits/echolalia attention deficit distractibility hyperactivity impulsivity anxiety hypersensitivity hand flapping and other repetitive movements impaired nonverbal behaviors (eye contact, etc.) impaired social interaction dense, immature brain cells
Gastrointestinal tract maturation	digestive problems allergies fungal overgrowth nutritional deficiencies leaky gut syndrome poor appetite

Metallothionein Functions	Autism Symptoms/Conditions
Regulation of metals (minerals and heavy metals)	skewed mineral ratios (high copper in ratio to low zinc) heavy metal toxicity (high levels of mercury, lead, cadmium, arsenic, and/or antimony) reactivity/sensitivity to heavy metals fungal overgrowth inability to process casein and gluten (heavy metals interfere with enzymes that break down casein and gluten)

protein wasn't working correctly. "When we did that, we came up with virtually every symptom of autism," he says. "We could explain everything from this one protein." The early abstract Dr. Walsh wrote on his findings concluded with the line: "These data suggest that an inborn error of metallothionein functioning may be a fundamental cause of autism."[147]

The Pfeiffer Treatment Center has long been expert at correcting disturbances in metal metabolism. "We've known for more than 25 years that two-thirds of people with behavior disorders have a metal metabolism problem," states Dr. Walsh. "And we've known for all that time that it was almost certainly a problem with metallothionein. The reason we were sure was because all of the metals that are managed by metallothionein are the very ones that are abnormal in these people."

For example, sociopaths—people with anti-social personality disorder—tend to have very low copper levels, he explains, as do people with obsessive-compulsive disorder. In the case of autism, it's a high copper-to-zinc ratio. Dr. Walsh emphasizes that it is the ratio that is important here. "We learned a while ago that you have to measure the ratio to get solid data. If you look at the individual elements, you can get fooled."

In treating the metallothionein problem in autistic patients, Dr. Walsh and the staff at PTC have discovered that, in some cases, it is a matter of a deficiency that can be corrected by supplementation with nutrients that promote metallothionein production. In others, supplementation does not correct the problem. In the former, the autism "may result from biochemical imbalances that impair MT [metallothionein] function rather than a direct genetic MT defect. This may explain the striking differences in autism patient outcomes," says Dr. Walsh.[148]

Environmental Triggers and Genetics

There are certain genes that regulate metallothionein and Dr. Walsh has launched research in collaboration with one of the world's leading experts on metallothionein genetics to determine which of those genes is implicated. "It's got us all excited," says Dr. Walsh, "because if this is correct, it means it may be possible to develop an inexpensive genetic test that can be given at birth to determine if there is a metal metabolism problem, and this might essentially prevent autism."

Two questions arise immediately in the discussion of autism as a genetic disease. One, how can autism be genetic since it is an epidemic disease at this point, and scientists agree that genetic disorders remain constant in the population and cannot be epidemic? Two, if it is genetic, how can it be prevented?

Many who say that autism is genetic deny the involvement of vaccines because environmental factors shouldn't affect the incidence of a genetic disease. Those who cannot ignore the correlation of the rise in autism with the increase in vaccinations eschew the genetic explanation in favor of environmental causality. Dr. Walsh states that both camps are partially correct. "What you have is a genetic disease, a genetic abnormality, that makes these particular children extraordinarily sensitive to the environment. So it's both genetic and environmental." Dr. Walsh concurs with those who believe that the increase both in the number of vaccines delivered in one shot and the total number of immunizations received has likely provided a widespread environmental trigger for these genetically at-risk children.

Another common explanation for the rise in autism is that the diagnosis is simply being dispensed more, misdiagnosis is therefore rampant, and the children who recover didn't actually have autism. Dr. Walsh dismisses this. The rise in autism is real, he states, as many elementary school teachers can testify. He cites one who told him that over 20 years of teaching, she only met one or two autistic kids, but now she meets one or two every year.

At PTC, there is some question in the diagnosis of only 10 or 20 percent of those who come to them, and some of those should have been diagnosed with autism and were not. "Some were diagnosed with childhood schizophrenia and some were labeled with obsessive compulsive disorder or seizure disorder, but the communication disorder [of autism] is so total usually, and the other symptoms are so striking, that it's not hard to diagnose in most cases."

So, *if autism is genetic, how can it be prevented?* Dr. *Walsh answers that two steps are important to take for prevention:* (1) *avoid the environmental triggers as much as possible and thereby sidestep the genetic susceptibility; and* (2) *supplement with nutrients that promote metallothionein.*

As for the view that a child who recovers after biochemical or other treatment can't have been truly autistic because that doesn't happen with a genetic disorder, Dr. Walsh counters, "Genetics doesn't mean hopeless or incurable. What genetics means, to me, is chemistry. Chemistry can be adjusted and corrected." He gives the example of someone with depression, in which a genetic component is involved (science acknowledges the role of genetics in depression). "Some people, whether with medication or with some other therapy, become free of depression. So does that mean it wasn't genetic? And they weren't really depressed?"

So, if autism is genetic, how can it be prevented? Dr. Walsh answers that two steps are important to take for prevention: (1) avoid the environmental triggers as much as possible and thereby sidestep the genetic susceptibility; and (2) supplement with nutrients that promote metallothionein (more on these later).

What are the specific triggers that are so problematic? Given the effects and functions of metallothionein, it can be postulated that heavy metal exposure and/or an assault on the immune system are major triggers in the development of autism. This explains why so many parents report that their child was fine until after a bout of flu or after immunizations (with or without mercury). Those may have been sufficient alone, depending upon the degree of vulnerability, or in combination with other environmental factors, to produce the disorder.

In the future, with a genetic test, children who are prone to autism can be identified before they've already got it, one hopes. Or, Dr. Walsh suggests, amniocentesis (a prenatal test) might be able to catch it even earlier. Then, the mother would know to avoid dental work involving mercury amalgam fillings, and to avoid flu shots. "They now give flu shots to many pregnant women in the U.S., and [the shots] may have 75 micrograms of mercury in them," observes Dr. Walsh. "That's not a good idea for these particular kids." Nor is a thimerosal-containing hepatitis B vaccine at birth, he adds.

If genetic testing revealed that a child had a tendency for autism, there are a number of preventive practices that could be implemented, says Dr. Walsh. The child would need to avoid all sources of toxic metals, including lead and cadmium. In addition to forgoing vaccinations with or without heavy metal preservatives, the child should drink only pure water. Well or tap water may contain high levels of minerals and heavy metals which, with a metal metabolism defect, the body can't process. Swimming pools and Jacuzzis may be treated with copper sulfate anti-algae agents, which would be another unwanted source of copper. The child would also need to avoid high-copper foods such as chocolate, carob, and shellfish, as well as copper-containing supplements and "enriched" foods.[149]

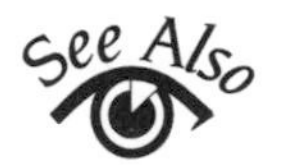

For information about alternative approaches to vaccination, see chapter 7.

The good news, notes Dr. Walsh, is that if a child doesn't develop autism by the age of three, "it's probably not going to happen, because by then the brain is sufficiently matured." It is the effects of a metal metabolism problem on a developing brain that produces autism, not only because of the body's inability to get rid of heavy metals, which are neurotoxic, but also because metallothionein, as mentioned above, is involved in the maturation of the brain.

Recoveries

For those children who already have autism, biochemical treatment can produce improvement; and in a few cases, complete recovery. The Pfeiffer Center has learned that when you give the supplements to get metallothionein working again and the child achieves homeostasis of copper and zinc levels in the blood, you can conclude that metallothionein is operational. Balancing metal levels is more difficult in autism, however, compared to ADHD and behavior disorders because of what appears to be the genetic defect in metallothionein function.

The Center's outcome studies indicate that 85 percent of autism patients achieve significant, long-lasting benefits, but only 5 to 10 percent of them are "what you would call 'miracles,' that is, autistic kids who become nearly free of symptoms," says Dr. Walsh. "It's such a beautiful thing when it happens. It's usually a very young child. If a person is 16 years old when we see him for the first time, I think the chance of one of those kinds of turnarounds is almost zero. But if you get a three-, four-, or five-year-old, they're the ones that may have the dramatic improvement."

One such case involved three-year-old twin girls, only one of whom was autistic. They were identical in appearance, although the parents weren't sure if they were actually identical versus fraternal twins. Their behavior made it easy to tell them apart, however. "You'd see the two of them together and you couldn't believe that they were twins," says Dr. Walsh. One was completely normal in her development, a charming, interactive child, while the other was nonverbal and displayed other typically autistic traits.

After two years of treatment, "I couldn't tell them apart," he reports. "I was startled because this little girl started talking to me and I called her by the wrong name. I thought it was her sister." It was the twin who had been diagnosed with autism, who no longer had autistic symptoms. When the parents sent the two girls to preschool, they didn't tell anybody at the school that one was autistic, and no one was the wiser.

Another of Dr. Walsh's cases of recovery is Marta, who was four years old when her parents brought her to PTC. Her problems had begun at around 18 months of age. A psychiatrist diagnosed her with severe autism, told the family that there was no cure, and recommended psychiatric medications and institutionalization. The family "would endure anything" rather than do that, recalls Dr. Walsh.

Her symptoms included running around in circles, no speech, diverse gaze, and no social relating—"she was just locked in her own little world." The family reported that she was also very sensitive to texture. She had to have certain kinds of clothes because she couldn't tolerate rough fabrics. Her sensitivity to textures extended to food, and there were few foods that she could stand to have in her mouth. Macaroni and cheese was about all she would eat. "That's one of the worst things she could eat," observes Dr. Walsh, "because it's loaded with gluten and casein. She had a nice case of casein/gluten allergy. Often, people crave the very thing that they're allergic to."

Marta's chemistry revealed the extraordinary copper/zinc imbalance present in most autistic patients. To rebalance these minerals, Marta was given a gradually increasing amount of zinc to stimulate the metallothionein protein, to help induce it into action, and a liberal amount of vitamin B_6. "The B_6 and zinc work together, and B_6 is directly involved in the synthesis of some of the neurotransmitters," explains Dr. Walsh.

Although the major problem was the severe metal metabolism disorder, Marta was also undermethylated. Methyl is one of the more common organic chemicals in the body; methyl groups are present in most enzymes and proteins. Methylation is the process by which methyl groups are added to a compound, making methyl available for the many reactions for which it is needed in the body.

For her methyl deficiency, Marta received the standard PTC supplement protocol of the amino acid methionine, calcium, magnesium, and vitamin B_6; these supplements increase methyl in the body and/or assist in methylation. Calcium is important because it helps lower histamine levels, but with undermethylation, histamine levels are high. Histamine is an essential protein metabolite found in all body tissues, and although most people associate it with allergies (it is what produces the runny nose, weepy eyes, and other signs of inflammation in an allergic reaction), in the brain histamine functions as a neurotransmitter. One category of schizophrenia is characterized by high histamine.[150]

Marta also had a history of gastrointestinal tract problems. She was already on a digestive enzyme, and Dr. Walsh continued that since the family reported that it helped. He gave her biotin (a member of the B-vitamin family), which is needed to maintain the integrity of the brush border of the intestines. The brush border is composed of many microvilli, the minute projections that vastly increase the surface of the intestines and give this border its velvety, brush-like appearance. Here, most nutrients are absorbed into the bloodstream.[151] If the brush border is compromised in some way, for example, by an overgrowth of *Candida*, nutrient absorption will be reduced. Thus, biotin supplementation or use of probiotics (beneficial intestinal bacteria; see following) can help increase absorption.

Marta's other supplements were the antioxidants vitamin C and vitamin E, and manganese. "Zinc, manganese, E, and C are all aimed at stimulating and inducing and promoting normal functioning of metallothionein," explains Dr. Walsh, adding that selenium and glutathione (a relative of glutamic acid, an amino acid) are also very useful nutrients for this purpose.

Four months later, when Marta came back for a follow-up, she was remarkably better. The family was overjoyed. She had started talking, with 15 or so words in her vocabulary. "The whole business of speech was beginning," Dr. Walsh notes. She no longer had behavioral upsets. "She used to melt down when she was unhappy, and that had disappeared."

These effects were accomplished with a treatment program consisting of supplements, and for her, "it just worked like a charm. I only wish that all autism patients had that kind of result," says Dr. Walsh.

At her annual checkup a year later—Marta was five years old by then—the family reported that she was in a regular kindergarten classroom, something they had been told would never happen, and doing very well. "She was also talking marvelously," Dr. Walsh remembers. Once she began talking, her family said, her vocabulary dramatically zoomed; they thought she was probably at grade level. At her next checkup a year later, the family announced that she was in a gifted classroom for very advanced students.

> **In Their Own Words**
>
> *"The fact that most doctors have not formally studied the effects of nutrition, food intolerance, and vitamins and minerals on health has generally led to a shunning of what this area of health practice may have to offer, and this is unfortunate....Since being treated for my own intolerances and deficiencies, I have been able to cope far better with the anxiety that set up a barrier to change, self-awareness, expression, and comprehension."*[152]
>
> —Donna Williams, author of *Nobody Nowhere: The Extraordinary Autobiography of an Autistic*

Marta is fourteen now, and no one would ever suspect that she had once been labeled severely autistic. As she entered puberty, her mother thought there was some slippage occurring and called Dr. Walsh. He recommended increasing the dosage of Marta's supplements to compensate for the weight gain and the growth spurt that accompanies the onset of puberty. "There's a bigger strain on metal metabolism then," he explains, "because hormonal changes result in copper elevation, and growth has a lot to do with zinc. So that's a really nasty combination for someone with this copper/zinc imbalance."

Having a copper/zinc imbalance doesn't necessarily mean a lifetime of taking supplements, however. "Once you get to the age of twenty and growth stops, a lot of pressure on this imbalance goes away," says Dr. Walsh. The cessation of growth takes away a lot of the need for zinc, which is used by the body for transcription, the copying of one cell to another when cells divide.

"Every time a cell divides, you lose zinc," he notes. This zinc drain ends when you stop growing. As a result, some patients find that they are able to get by with lower doses or no doses at all. "We occasionally run into people who found that they didn't have to do our treatment at all after age 20." Marta, however, will probably need supplements throughout her life to counteract the genetic disorder by promoting metallothionein. Regardless, she is one of the lucky PTC recoveries.

Dr. Walsh is careful to say that such cases are not the norm. "We have a number of people who become completely free of symptoms and it's exciting, but I wouldn't want to give the impression that everyone gets that much better. . . . [U]sually what we see is a nice, partial improvement." While improvement in 85 percent of those who seek treatment is an impressive percentage, it is not good enough for Dr. Walsh. "If an autistic child has wild behavior, doesn't talk, and doesn't socialize, and you correct the behavior completely, that family is thrilled. But the child is still autistic. Or say another child who is autistic has no speech, can't do parallel play, and all of that, and after you start treating the child, the child begins to talk. Again, the family may be thrilled, it has a nice improvement, but the child is still autistic."

In behavior disorders, depression, and even schizophrenia, PTC's success rates are much higher, and treatment leaves a lot of these patients completely without symptoms, he notes. "We do well with our [autistic] patients—I think we do as well as anybody—but in my view, we need to do much better." With the refinement of treatment, based on their recent metallothionein findings, that is likely to be the case.

A Closer Look at the Metallothionein Connection

As cited in the sidebar on pages 115–116, the effects of a metallothionein defect correlate with the symptoms and conditions associated with autism. The following briefly looks at the reasons behind some of these corrrelations.

Weakened Immunity

As metallothionein is required for the immune system, one could make a case that the viruses in vaccines, given in close succession and often with multiple viruses in one immunization, gradually weaken the immune system, and eventually knock it down. "It could be a cumulative effect," notes Dr. Walsh. The vaccine MMR may be the final straw in the viral overload, he adds, as this is the vaccine most often cited by parents as the one after which their child developed autistic symptoms. The fact that MMR is a mercury-free injection supports the conjecture that viral overload is the issue in this case. "I think it's a likely possibility, but unproven," concludes Dr. Walsh.

Heavy Metal Toxicity

Metallothionein is crucial to the body in regulating and coping with toxic metals. For example, if mercury enters the body, metallothionein is supposed to become mercury-metallothionein. "It sort of envelopes the mercury," explains Dr. Walsh. This protein "has a tremendous affinity for mercury, far beyond any other chemical in the body." To this end, there is a lot of metallothionein in the liver and in the intestinal tract, "so whether you would inhale or swallow that mercury or lead or cadmium, most of it would interact and be bound to metallothionein, which would protect the rest of the body from harm."

If this system is working well, you can handle even a significant dose of mercury; it will simply be excreted from the body. But with autism, this doesn't seem to be the case. "If you postulate that these kids have an inborn or genetic error of metallothionein or something that disables that protein, you would expect that they would be incredibly sensitive to toxic metals," states Dr. Walsh, "and that's what tens of thousands of families are reporting."

Gastrointestinal and Nervous System Impairment

Metallothionein is involved in the maturation of the brain and the gastrointestinal tract, as well as the formation and regulation of nerve cells including brain cells. If the metallothionein system is not working, you would expect that the brain and the GI tract might not fully mature, states Dr. Walsh. Many of the symptoms of autism are related to brain and nervous system function. Digestive complaints, such as candidiasis and food allergies/sensitivities, are commonly associated with autism.

Dr. Walsh explains the mechanism behind two food sensitivities widely evidenced in autistic children: gluten and casein. "If you have mercury or lead in the gut, and you do not have metallothionein there to disable the toxic substance, the most likely place for it to go is to chemicals called sulfhydral groups." A combination of sulphur and hydrogen, these groups have tremendous power to bind to mercury, lead, and cadmium, but especially mercury, notes Dr. Walsh.

Among the sulfhydral groups in the intestines are the enzymes that break down casein and gluten. Toxins interfere with their function. In addition, the manufacture of these enzymes requires zinc. With the severe zinc depletion common to children with autism, production will necessarily suffer.

So without metallothionein to deal with toxins and supply zinc, the enzymes will be in low concentration and prone to disabling by toxins. "You would expect these kids to have extraordinary problems with unprocessed casein and gluten, which is exactly what people are finding over and over."

An Overview of Biochemical Therapy for Autism

As stated earlier, biochemical therapy is based on the tenet of individualized treatment, given that each person's biochemistry is unique. That said, children with autism often require similar treatment because they suffer from many of the same biochemical imbalances and associated conditions, such as intestinal problems. While dosages may vary, depending upon body weight and degree of deficiency or imbalance, many of these children need the same basic supplements.

Since the digestive tract of autistic children is usually not functioning very well, the supplements that comprise the core of treatment may not be absorbed well. About 85 percent of all autistics have malabsorption and gastrointestinal tract problems,

The Four Types of Metallothionein

A factor that makes the reversal of a metallothionein defect more complicated is that there are four kinds of metallothionein, designated metallothionein (or MT) -1, -2, -3, and -4. Metallothionein-3 is only in the brain, and metallothionein-4 is only in the upper gastrointestinal tract, while metallothionein-1 and -2 are in every cell throughout the body. Further, metallothionein easily gets to the brain, Dr. Walsh explains, but to function there it needs to be bound to glutamate (a salt of glutamic acid, the only amino acid metabolized by the brain).

The upshot of this discussion, according to Dr. Walsh, is that "the road map for determining the way to properly treat autism, to medically, clinically treat and balance the chemical imbalances, you need to know which of these metallothioneins is affected." For example, if it's MT-4, you would focus on correcting the gastrointestinal tract. If it's MT-3, you might focus on brain chemistry, especially glutamate chemistry. If it's 1 and 2, you might focus on glutathione and achieving homeostasis of the blood. At the present time, with no way to identify which of the metallothioneins are involved, "We aren't sure what is the best direction to focus this treatment," Dr. Walsh says. "Identifying the autism gene(s) may lead to greatly improved autism therapies."

compared to about 10 percent of children with attention deficit, according to Dr. Walsh. So, when someone with autism is first seen at the Pfeiffer Center, "we try to set up their system to get ready for our treatment," he says. Since it takes about a month to get all the laboratory results back, establish a diagnosis in biochemical terms (identify imbalances), and design treatment, probiotic supplementation is instituted immediately in individuals with gastrointestinal symptoms. These friendly bacteria can help reduce fungal overgrowth and restore intestinal integrity. To assist digestion, special formulations of digestive enzymes that survive stomach acids may also be recommended.

As a further aid to healing the digestive system and making treatment more effective, Dr. Walsh recommends the casein/gluten-free diet because these substances are problematic for most autistic children and the diet has proven beneficial. "We think every autistic deserves at least a trial of that diet," he says, adding the hopeful news that it may only be a temporary measure. "They may not need to do it once we get the metallothionein part corrected."

Since the digestive tract of autistic children is usually not functioning very well, the supplements that comprise the core of treatment may not be absorbed well. About 85 percent of all autistics have malabsorption and gastrointestinal tract problems, compared to about 10 percent of children with attention deficit, according to Dr. Walsh.

At PTC, they have learned that the route to success seems to be "to do whatever you can with the gastrointestinal tract and with toxic substances early. We call it metabolic priming, getting the system primed," says Dr. Walsh. In addition to correcting metal metabolism, which has far-reaching effects on many systems in the body, other problems may need to be addressed. For example, as in Marta's case, the person may be undermethylated or there may be essential fatty acid, or other, abnormalities. "For autism, we have to focus primarily on the GI tract and metallothionein, but if there is something else wrong, we have to address that, too."

Since there is no commercial test to measure metallothionein in the body, PTC relies on the ratio of blood levels of zinc, copper, and ceruloplasmin (a substance in the blood to which copper attaches) as indicators of malfunction of this protein. After metabolic priming, treatment for this malfunction includes zinc, manganese, selenium, vitamin B_6, vitamin C, vitamin E, glutathione, and the fourteen amino acid constituents of metallothionein. Often, a liquid form of the desired supplements is used, since many children have trouble swallowing capsules. A pharmacy that does liquid compounding of vitamins and minerals prepares a compound of the correct amounts and nutrients needed by an individual.

Once metallothionein is functioning normally again, in many cases, "the body just naturally takes over and you get rid of the toxic substances, you get homeostasis of copper and zinc, the gut problems usually disappear, the food sensitivities may disappear, and the body is protected against future toxic exposures," says Dr. Walsh. "The primary nutrient needed in the formation of metallothionein is zinc, so if you're extraordinarily zinc deficient, that will disable the system."

As the supplement program gradually brings the metallothionein protein into proper function, detoxification gets going again. The emphasis here is on *gradual.* "We learned long ago that we don't dare suddenly bring it to life," Dr. Walsh explains. "Because if that happens, the metallothionein works so well that it suddenly causes an excessive amount of toxic substances in the tissues to be released all at once. And that could cause nasty symptoms and stress the kidneys." To prevent this, the dosages of the supplements that stimulate metallothionein are slowly increased over time.

As noted previously, before you undertake detoxification, you need to be sure that the liver and kidneys are healthy. Testing liver enzymes and kidney function is part of PTC's standard medical testing. Dr. Walsh has found that compromised liver and kidney health can be avoided in the autistic population through careful monitoring of treatment by a physician.

The HRIPTC database of 503 autistic individuals revealed that a majority had elevated levels of lead, cadmium, arsenic, antimony, and/or mercury. (While some people are pointing to high aluminum as a factor in autism, Dr. Walsh's data shows no evidence of that.) "Almost all these kids have higher toxic levels than other kids," he says. "The reason is that, with this metallothionein malfunction, they will not be able to handle the kind of toxic exposures that we all get every day." He cites typical daily exposures: 1 microgram of mercury per day just from breathing; 20 micrograms per day from food, with that number rising to 40 or 50 micrograms per day if tuna is consumed.

The initial treatment to restore metallothionein function may not be sufficient to detoxify the body. In fact, says Dr. Walsh, "From our experience with all these thousands of people we've treated for metal metabolism disorders, very often you don't get the copper/zinc completely balanced unless you give them cysteine [on its own]."

The mention of this amino acid, which is the primary ingredient of metallothionein (twenty out of the sixty-one amino acid components of metallothionein are cysteine), may raise alarm in those who are acquainted with its detoxification application to autism. "There are a lot of people in the field that feel it should be forever banned from use for autism," states Dr. Walsh. "The reason is they've tried it and they get these horrible reactions since it works too fast and causes the toxins to be dumped too quickly." That can produce a number of unpleasant symptoms.

There is no cause for alarm with cysteine as long as it is used correctly, states Dr. Walsh. "Correctly" means that some level of metal detoxification has already occurred, as is the case when metallothionein function has been restored gradually. "We don't use cysteine for the first four months, because it works too fast," he says, explaining that it works so rapidly because it has a great affinity for metals. Administered after the body has had a chance to detoxify for a while, cysteine—along with zinc and glutathione—is the most effective nutrient for getting rid of excess copper and heavy metals, states Dr. Walsh.

As for mercury detoxification protocols practiced by other doctors, Dr. Walsh has heard a number of these doctors speak of a phenomenon that mystifies them in their treatment of autistic children. While the children exhibit remarkable improvements following mercury detoxification, the doctors report that the benefits soon disappear.

"The benefits they are seeing may not result from mercury leaving," says Dr. Walsh, "but from improved antioxidant status from bringing copper down." As most autistics exhibit a severe copper-overload condition, "you would expect that in a day or two you would see a nice improvement. But chelation therapy is ineffective at correcting the copper overload or metallothionein dysfunction, and there's no protection against future toxic exposures." As a result, when copper levels rise again, symptoms return.

Pyroluria and Autism

A disorder called pyroluria is operational in a small percentage of those with autism. They may have this alone or in combination with other imbalances. Dr. Walsh notes that the autistic children who reverse the fastest and most completely with treatment seem to be the ones with pyroluria. "That's a disorder that can correct in two to four days—and those are the biggest miracles."

A pyrrole is a basic chemical structure used in the manufacture of heme, which is what makes the blood red. Pyroluria is a genetic disorder in pyrrole chemistry, characterized by an overproduction of kryptopyrroles (hidden pyrroles) during the synthesis of hemoglobin (the iron-rich component of the blood that carries oxygen). As kryptopyrroles bind with vitamin B_6 and zinc, which are then excreted in the urine, this leads to deficiencies in those nutrients. People with pyroluria may have low levels of the neurotransmitter serotonin as vitamin B_6 is needed for its synthesis.[153] Pyroluria is known to scientists and physicians with a biochemical orientation for its connection to schizophrenia.

It may be connected to autism as well, according to Dr. Walsh. "The pyrrole disorder apparently can cause either autism or schizophrenia," he says. The encouraging point in this is that pyroluria is easily treated (mainly with zinc and B_6 supplements), and is the most reversible kind of autism. Dr. Walsh postulates that metallothionein in pyroluric autistics is disabled by the severe zinc deficiency associated with the chemical imbalance rather than a genetic defect, which explains its reversibility. His clinical experience supports that view.

Jason: Close Monitoring

The following case illustrates the importance of continuing to treat every patient individually, regardless of how standard the initial biochemical treatment for autism may be.

Jason was diagnosed with autism when he was two years old. "The family was told that he probably should be institutionalized. He was raging and wild, had lost his speech, and had digestive problems," recalls Dr. Walsh, who has been treating Jason for a year with PTC's typical program to restore metallothionein function.

He reports that Jason is doing "marvelously well," talking normally and no longer having the meltdowns and behavior tantrums so common prior to treatment. "Instead of looking worried all the time, he seems so sweet and cuddly now, smiling all the time."

Recently, the boy's father reported that Jason had been having digestive upsets, which were accompanied by a return of his other symptoms. At those times, he could see his son heading downhill. Jason's temper would start to build and his eye contact socialization would degenerate. The father saw an exact correlation between the return of the autistic symptoms and Jason's bowel status, such as when he had a bout of diarrhea. "We thought we had his digestive problems nicely overcome—he seemed to be 95 percent without symptoms—but it looks like part of [the autism] comes back every time his GI tract is disturbed," says Dr. Walsh.

Retesting revealed that Jason's copper/zinc imbalance had gotten large again. Dr. Walsh believes the episodes are a reflection of the degree to which treatment is keeping Jason's chemistry balanced. "[Chemistry] changes with time," he explains. "It changes with stress level; it changes with general health; it changes with diet. It could be caused by something as simple as catching the flu." Also, with young patients like Jason, you have to keep on top of their chemistry because they grow so fast and dosages need to be changed accordingly, he says. In Jason's case, an increase in his supplement dosages seems to have ameliorated the digestive problems and the reversion they produced.

"It's a vicious circle when you have a problem with your GI tract," says Dr. Walsh. Food and supplements are not processed as efficiently, and you get fewer nutrients from what you are swallowing. When your nutrient intake begins to deteriorate, then everything goes."

In Jason's case, closer monitoring seems to be advisable. While most other children only come in for annual checkups, Dr. Walsh thinks Jason may need to come four or five times a year. Although he is thriving, "he is still more sensitive than the average person," says Dr. Walsh. "Complete recovery is likely. He's been there before, so we know we've got our hand on the right lever. We just have to keep adjusting those doses."

David: Treatment at Twenty-Five

As many practitioners in this book state, treatment is most effective when begun early, the earlier the better. Nevertheless, biochemical therapy can also have benefits for adults with autism, as the following case illustrates.

David came to PTC at the age of twenty-five. Dr. Walsh describes him as "a tall, slender, quite hyper young man, with very little meaningful speech," and notes that he had difficulty in public because he looked peculiar and acted strangely. He had been diagnosed with autism when he was five or six years old, and his parents had taken him to many experts, but little change resulted. The family sought Dr. Walsh's help because David's rages were getting worse. He would go into wild, physical rages and tear apart the house, according to his parents. They said that the inside of their house looked as if a bomb had hit it. The parents knew that PTC's best success rates were with younger children, but they had to do something.

The treatment helped David quite a bit. He got "considerably better," according to Dr. Walsh. His violent episodes disappeared, and his general health improved significantly. He had always been sick a lot, and that was no longer the case after treatment.

Biochemically, he was very like Marta (see "Recoveries"). Along with having the metal metabolism problem, he was another of those high histamine, undermethylated people. Dr. Walsh notes that high histamine and undermethylation are both associated with a tendency toward ritualism, perseveration, and repetitive movements and activities. Undermethylation, in particular, is associated with obsessive-compulsive disorders, as is autism.

As David's biochemistry was so similar to Marta's, he got the same treatment, with the dosages of the various supplements adjusted according to his metabolic weight factor. This is a method of calculating dosages based on metabolism, Dr. Walsh explains. It is far more accurate than figuring dosage as a mere percentage of the standard 160-pound person. The latter method results in underdosing small people and overdosing big people. If you have someone who is 320 pounds, for example, it is not correct to give them twice the dose of a 160-pound person, says Dr. Walsh.

Reversing undermethylation is "a slow, gradual process that takes four to six months to complete," he says, "although supplementation with SAMe can speed up the process." (SAMe, which stands for S-adenosylmethionine, is manufactured in the body from the amino acid methionine, and is involved in many metabolic processes, including the production of brain chemicals. SAMe is available as a supplement.) In addition to his other problems, David was also very low in serotonin, a neurotransmitter involved in mood regulation. The treatment worked to raise those levels as well but, again, it was a slow process.

David was one of those patients with whose treatment results Dr. Walsh was not satisfied. Yes, David was healthier and his meltdowns had stopped—he was no longer tearing the house apart. The family was very happy with that improvement. "But he still had the lack of socialization, and he still wasn't talking much better. So it's a nice partial improvement, but to me it was disappointing," states Dr. Walsh. It is clear from the way he says this that his disappointment is on David's behalf and stems from his desire for everyone to be free of this painful disorder.

The Future

It is Dr. Walsh's dedication to ending the epidemic of autism that led him to go public with his findings before publishing them in a scientific journal. By doing this, he risked someone else running with the idea and beating him into publication, thus claiming the credit for discovery of a universal metallothionein disorder as the cause of autism.

"We decided that if this could lead to early prevention, we had to release this information before it was published. We felt that to do the standard scientific thing of writing up the results, submitting it to a journal, waiting eight months or a year to be published when there are thirty-five new cases of autism every day in America—we're talking about thousands and thousands of families—we couldn't sleep at night if we did that."

Dr. Walsh hopes that by putting the information out to the scientific community, it will attract a lot of attention among clinicians and researchers and more people will get involved in investigating the metallothionein hypothesis. For those who are skeptical, Dr. Walsh tells them that if they sample the blood of a few autistic children, they will find the same thing as he did. "Then if they investigate what metallothionein's functions are, they'll quickly come to the same conclusions. When you have 500 people and almost all of them have the same problem, that's hard to explain."

He notes that metallothionein dysfunction as the cause of autism also explains why four times more boys than girls develop the condition. Estrogen and progesterone, the "female" hormones, induce metallothionein production and protect against environmental insult. With a genetic weakness in metallothionein, boys will be less protected than girls.

Dr. Walsh's hopes for what research can accomplish extend beyond the ability to identify who is vulnerable to autism, so they can then avoid the known environmental triggers. He speaks of the possibility of autism reversal. If metallothionein itself is genetically defective, with so much metallothionein in the intestinal tract, "one might be able to reverse autism without having to target any interior organs."

Here, Dr. Walsh is referring to the dangerous procedure of targeting organs for alteration of DNA defects. It would be a lot safer, he notes, to reverse the metallothionein defect just within the intestines. "If in fact it is metallothionein, gene therapy may be capable of safely reversing autism. That's something that is a possibility and we are moving as fast as we can, working as hard as we can."

Meanwhile, Dr. Walsh and his colleagues are making changes in the treatment of autism at PTC, based on what they've learned about metallothionein. "We constantly try to improve it," he says, adding that an outcome study to test efficacy of the revised program is pending. "It will probably take us another year until we have people who have been treated long enough to do a proper outcome study and measure results."

Dr. Walsh can state unequivocally at this time that "for an autistic child to reach his full potential," metallothionein dysfunction needs to be addressed.

As for his metallothionein model of autism, Dr. Walsh concludes, "I certainly hope for the benefit of the families that it is correct. Autism is a tragic disease." He can state unequivocally at this time, however, that "for an autistic child to reach his full potential," metallothionein dysfunction needs to be addressed.

7 Homeopathy: Constitutional Treatment, Vaccine Clearing, and an Alternative to Vaccines

Homeopathy has strong application for autism in a number of ways. Special homeopathic preparations called nosodes have been used to great effect in clearing adverse vaccine reactions from the body, as case studies in this chapter illustrate. Other beneficial applications include constitutional treatment, nosodes as an alternative to vaccines, and the treatment of childhood illnesses with homeopathic remedies. This chapter first looks at constitutional treatment, which is also known as classical homeopathy.

What Is Homeopathy?

To understand homeopathy, it is helpful to consider the derivation of the word as well as that of allopathy, both of which were coined by the father of homeopathy, Dr. Samuel Hahnemann, in the late 1700s. A German physician and chemist who became increasingly frustrated with conventional medical practice, Dr. Hahnemann devoted himself to developing a safer, more effective approach to medicine. The result was homeopathy, which arose out of his discovery that illness can be treated by giving the patient a dilution of a plant that produces symptoms resembling those of the illness when given to a healthy person.

This principle, "let likes be cured with likes," became known as the Law of Similars. Dr. Hahnemann named this system of healing homeopathy, a combination of the Greek *homoios* (similar) and *pathos* (suffering). At the same time, he dubbed conventional medicine allopathy, which means "opposite suffering," to reflect that model's approach of treating illness by giving an antidote to the symptoms, a medicine that produces the opposite effect from what the patient is suffering. (A laxative for constipation is an illustration of the allopathic approach; it produces diarrhea.)[154]

Homeopathic remedies can be employed as simple remedies to address a certain transitory ailment or as constitutional remedies to address the whole cluster of physical, psychological, and emotional characteristics—the constitution—of an individual patient. A constitutional remedy works to restore balance and thus health on all levels.

Homeopathic remedies are prepared through a process of dilution of plant substances, which results in a "potentized" remedy, one that contains the energy imprint of the plant rather than its biochemical components. This is why homeopathy falls into the category of energy medicine; it works on an energetic level to effect change in all aspects of a person and restore balance to the whole.

Paradoxically, the higher the number of dilutions, the greater the potency and the effects of the remedy. Thus the higher the potency number, the more powerful the remedy. Remedies used to treat a transitory condition are usually 6C, 12C, or 30C, relatively low-potency remedies. A constitutional remedy is often a 1M potency, which means it has been diluted a thousand times.

Constitutional Treatment of Autism

Classical or constitutional homeopathic treatment is distinct from the use of homeopathic nosodes (explained later in the chapter) or remedies for acute symptoms in that it employs a single remedy that addresses the particular and unique mental, emotional, and physical composition of an individual. Judyth Reichenberg-

Ullman, N.D., M.S.W., a homeopathic and naturopathic physician who practices in Edmonds, Washington, explains it this way: "Each child, or adult, is much like a jigsaw puzzle. Once all of the pieces are assembled in their proper places, an image emerges that is distinct from other puzzles. It is the task of a homeopath to recognize that image and to match it to the corresponding image of one specific homeopathic medicine."[155]

The homeopath makes that match by considering the person's behaviors, feelings, attitudes, beliefs, likes, dislikes, physical symptoms, prenatal and birth history, family medical history, eating and sleeping patterns, and even dreams and fears.[156] By giving the remedy whose qualities match this unique cluster most closely, the homeopathic principle of "like cures like" is put into operation and the remedy works to restore the person to balance. People may have one constitutional remedy that is their match throughout their life, or it may change over time and a different constitutional remedy might then be required.

Homeopathy does not prescribe according to diagnostic labels, but rather according to the complete picture of the individual. Thus, two children with autism may require two entirely different remedies.

A single dose of a constitutional remedy is sometimes all that is needed at first. When the remedy is the correct one for an individual, changes can begin relatively quickly, within two to five weeks after taking the dose. (Some people experience changes in the first day, or even within hours.) If there are no changes within five weeks, that may indicate that it is not the proper remedy. A remedy continues to work over time, anywhere from four months to a year or longer. Repeat doses may be necessary if there is a relapse of symptoms, or sometimes a different remedy may be called for, as was true for Tyler in the case study to follow.

Due to the way homeopathic remedies work, it is important to continue treatment for one to two years at least, states Dr. Reichenberg-Ullman. This does not mean frequent appointments with your homeopath, however. In fact, she says, "In cases of children with significant developmental problems, we have found that it is often better to allow at least two months to elapse between visits in order to evaluate the full extent of progress."[157] As time goes by, the number of visits can decrease further.

While certain substances (notably coffee, menthol, camphor, and eucalyptus) can antidote homeopathic remedies, prescription medications such as Ritalin do not interfere with their function, and vice versa. (Topical steroids, antibiotics, and antifungals are to be avoided, however, and oral antibiotics and cortisone products should only be used in consultation with your homeopath.[158]) Thus, parents can pursue homeopathic treatment for their child, even if they do not want to stop the regulatory medications.

Some parents opt for homeopathy from the beginning, before starting their child on drugs. Others come to treatment later and, in consultation with their prescribing physician, elect to replace the drugs with homeopathy. Still others continue the drugs until it is clear by the change in the child that the homeopath has found the correct remedy. "[O]nce the right homeopathic medicine has been prescribed, the conventional drugs are often not necessary," notes Dr. Reichenberg-Ullman.[159]

In her practice, Dr. Reichenberg-Ullman has found that children with significant developmental delay can benefit from homeopathic treatment.

The Benefits of Homeopathic Treatment

Dr. Reichenberg-Ullman cites the following benefits of constitutional homeopathic treatment.[160] Homeopathy:

- treats the whole person
- treats the root of the problem
- treats each person as an individual
- uses natural, nontoxic medicines
- is considered safe and does not have the side effects of Ritalin and other prescription drugs
- heals physical, mental, and emotional symptoms
- uses medicines, one dose of which works for months or years rather than hours
- uses inexpensive medicines
- is cost effective.

"Children who are developmentally disabled, with or without behavioral problems, can sometimes achieve amazing strides in behavior, coping skills, and learning abilities."[161]

The following cases from her patient files illustrate the wide scope of changes possible with homeopathic treatment of autistic children. In Justin's case, this treatment allowed him to avoid being put on prescription medications. Tyler's story demonstrates how homeopathic remedies can be used safely and concurrently with medications such as Ritalin and Dexedrine, and enable the child to be weaned off these drugs.

Justin: Asperger's Disorder

When his parents consulted Dr. Reichenberg-Ullman, Justin was seven years old and had received a diagnosis of Asperger's disorder.‡ His mother reported that he was "in his own world," and was limited in his ability to function appropriately around others. His speech had been delayed and, until he was four years old, his vocabulary consisted of only 20 words. He was always different from other children—singing to himself, seemingly oblivious to social cues, and acting without apparent awareness. He avoided eye contact and tended toward repetitious speech and perseveration on minute details, particularly of his computer games. His attention span was short, and his distractibility was creating problems for his teachers.

Justin was a pacer and also displayed aggressive tendencies. He had a very loud voice, was prone to screaming, and suffered from impulsive, out-of-control moods in which he became threatening and even physically violent. In one such mood, he attacked his brother and wrapped a radio cord around his brother's neck. In between these moods, he was helpful and loving toward his

---

‡This case study adapted, by permission of Judyth Reichenberg-Ullman, N.D., from *Ritalin-Free Kids: Safe and Effective Homeopathic Medicine for ADHD, and Other Behavioral and Learning Problems,* by Judyth Reichenberg-Ullman, N.D., M.S.W., and Robert Ullman, N.D. (Roseville, California: Prima Health, 2000), pages 212–215.

family, his parents reported. He craved attention from adults and would do whatever he could to get his parents to stop talking to each other and pay attention to him.

In response to Dr. Reichenberg-Ullman's inquiries about the pregnancy, Justin's mother revealed that she went through a rocky time with Justin's father while pregnant with Justin, and she feared that he might abandon her as a previous boyfriend had done. In fact, she held the deep-seated belief that it was inevitable that her partner would leave her because she was not good enough.

All of this contributed to the picture of Justin, which indicated the constitutional remedy that would be a match for him. The physical complaints that completed the picture included "an itchy butt," a tendency toward loose stools, and an outbreak of hives that lasted for nine months after his MMR immunization.

Another homeopath had treated Justin with *Sulphur*, which produced partial improvement in his condition. "*Sulphur* is an excellent match for the tendency to be in his own world, obliviousness to social cues, and his mother's feeling of being scorned, which, we believe, could have affected Justin," says Dr. Reichenberg-Ullman. However, she determined that the more appropriate remedy for him was *Baryta sulphuricum* (barium sulphate). "Barium covers Justin's shyness, delayed development, and awkwardness." The sulphur component of the remedy offers the previously mentioned benefits.

After two-and-a-half months, Justin was more aware and less in his own world, according to his mother. He was less wild and unruly, was able to socialize more, and seemed to be developing a sense of empathy. His spelling had also gotten better. In the following months, the improvements maintained, and he had fewer flarings of temper, stopped hurting other people, and his threats became less frequent. He also stopped pacing and could engage more in two-way conversations.

One year and four months after starting treatment, Justin's parents raved about their "new and improved child." The only remedy he needed was *Baryta sulphuricum,* which he has taken six times to date. He has not needed any psychiatric medications, which are a common prescription in cases of Asperger's disorder.

***Tyler*: Off the Drugs**

Tyler's mother contacted Dr. Reichenberg-Ullman after reading her book *Ritalin-Free Kids.*[§] She hoped homeopathy might help her autistic son, then 10 years old.

While the pregnancy was uneventful, Tyler's entry into the world was a bit traumatic. He was two weeks overdue when his mother's water broke, amidst a blizzard. The one obstetrician on call for two hospitals was already attending to a delivery at the other hospital when his mother arrived on the maternity ward at the second hospital. Tyler's pulse became weak during the wait, the doctor got involved in a car accident on his way from the other hospital, and Tyler had to be delivered via cesarean section.

He was rather flaccid compared to other babies, and he was unable to settle down and slept poorly. When he was three months old, his mother stopped breast-feeding, and at six months old, she placed him in day care and went back to work. Tyler had repeated ear infections and bouts of conjunctivitis, and two episodes of bronchitis.

"Tyler's parents always felt there was something different about him," states Dr. Dr. Reichenberg-Ullman. He showed little interest in people and was fascinated with light switches and buttons. At two years old, his development seemed to be regressing. He was demanding and restless, would not stay in his crib, screamed for what he wanted, and insisted on being held or accompanied around the house. In terms of speech development, he spoke only one word at a time, typically to demand something.

His mother reported that taking him anywhere "was a nightmare." She had to watch him constantly both in public and at home. In the supermarket, he would run six aisles away in a matter of

---

[§]This case study adapted, by permission of Judyth Reichenberg-Ullman, N.D., from *Ritalin-Free Kids: Safe and Effective Homeopathic Medicine for ADHD, and Other Behavioral and Learning Problems*, by Judyth Reichenberg-Ullman, N.D., M.S.W., and Robert Ullman, N.D. (Roseville, California: Prima Health, 2000), pages 215-220.

seconds. At home, one of Tyler's favorite occupations was to stuff objects into electric sockets; he was able to remove safety plugs faster than his mother could. He also had a penchant for hiding things, notably by dropping them in the heating vents. There was little relief from the vigilance of watching Tyler because he only slept four to six hours a night and, once he was a year old, never took a nap.

When Tyler was three and a half, his family moved and his behavior became more wild and erratic. At his new day care, the difference between Tyler and the other children was more apparent. His behavior was completely dissimilar and he kept apart from them, not joining in their play. Unfortunately, he was misdiagnosed at this point with ADHD, a label that stayed with him for the next four years.

Tyler's vocabulary was not increasing; he could not recognize letters or colors, did not participate in school projects, and was slow in learning. He did not respond to attempts to get his attention, and he tended to walk on his tiptoes, two classic symptoms of autism. His behavior became worse, and he began to hit, bite, and slap his classmates. He would not cooperate with his teacher. These developments prompted a psychiatrist to put him on Ritalin, which produced some improvement in his behavior. Tyler's parents consulted Dr. Reichenberg-Ullman for treatment at this time.

Although in a regular classroom, Tyler was then classified as learning disabled in some subjects. Tyler's teachers reported that he was quite anxious about keeping up with the other children and was easily set off, at which point he would cry, scream, rage, and pace hysterically. He tended to insist he was right about something even if he was clearly wrong. Along with the Ritalin, the psychiatrist then put him on Dexedrine, an amphetamine that is used to control hyperactivity in children. When Tyler didn't take his medications, he was antsy, fidgety, walked in circles, and roamed around the classroom talking to himself.

Tyler not only avoided interacting, but he didn't even seem to see the other children and turned his back on adults attempting to assist him. While his reasoning skills were good and he could aptly do equations and engage in complicated games, he could not generalize learning nor easily make the transition from one activity to another. Body language eluded him completely.

Among his quirks were a hatred of water, particularly getting his face wet, which he had evinced since he was a baby. Haircuts and combing were painful to him. He walked in his sleep and still suffered from nightmares, which had formerly been night terrors that left him inconsolable. He was fearless in other areas, however, walking to the edge of a cliff with no hesitation or uneasiness, for example. Tyler demonstrated considerable mechanical ability, once even figuring out how to stop an airport luggage carousel. When flashlight batteries disappeared at his house, his parents knew who had taken them.

The homeopathic remedy Dr. Reichenberg-Ullman gave him was *Helium*, indicated for children who are nonreactive, unapproachable, and distant. "It is curious that helium, as a substance, possesses no electrical resistance and, therefore, climbs up the walls of containers as if to defy gravity," she observes. "Just like Tyler when he fearlessly approached steep precipices."

In the space of two months, significant changes occurred. Tyler began to pay attention to making friends, the walking around in circles decreased, and he began to narrate information to his parents in great detail. His sleepwalking ended, and he reported dreams of conversing with people. He was better able to switch from one task to another and could comb his hair without pain. He was also more gentle with the family dog, whom he had formerly tended to squeeze too tightly when he was frustrated.

Almost six months later, Tyler had maintained his improved impulse control and was still not sleepwalking. He was even more engaged with other children, and his verbal skills were better. In the next year, Tyler's gains continued in all areas at home and at school. His mother assessed his impulsivity as "almost 100 percent better." He did not get frustrated as easily and was more adaptable to life in general. He no longer pushed buttons obsessively, as on the television remote control, and made it through barbershop haircuts without his former screaming.

At school, Tyler was still in a learning-disabilities class for reading and writing, but at the end of the year he was on the honor roll. The teachers regarded his scores as "admirable for any child." If a subject interested him, he was quite verbal. He also was able to identify most of his classmates by name.

"Tyler's parents had chosen to keep him on medications despite his improvement with homeopathy," says Dr. Reichenberg-Ullman. "After a year, however, they realized that it no longer made any difference when he forgot to take his Dexedrine." They began to wean him off it. At the consultation at that point, Tyler initiated conversation with Dr. Reichenberg-Ullman for the first time, chatting about his move to a mainstream classroom and how it didn't bother him much anymore if other kids teased him. His mother added that he required less assistance in the classroom, handled his responsibilities better, and turned in his schoolwork promptly.

Helium was the only homeopathic remedy he needed for the first two years of treatment. At that point, he was vastly improved. The main problem was that he tended to vegetate on the couch after school, more interested in his Power Rangers than in people. He also remained disinterested in bathing. Dr. Reichenberg-Ullman gave him a dose of *Sulphur*, which would further peer interaction and the completion of assignments, and help him to be less in his own world. When Tyler began to relapse six months later, she repeated the *Sulphur*. His condition improved again.

"Usually we find that a single homeopathic medicine repeated at infrequent intervals is most effective," she notes. In Tyler's case, he benefited from three remedies: *Helium*, *Sulphur*, and *Helleborus* (black hellebore). The third remedy enabled him "to take a further step toward appropriate social interaction." Overall, Tyler's mother estimated that her son improved 75 to 80 percent as a result of homeopathic treatment.

Homeopathic Nosodes

Isopathy is the term for the therapeutic administration of nosodes, which are homeopathic preparations of a pathogen. Many homeopaths include the use of nosodes under the rubric of homeopathy, but others prefer the term isopathy as a more accurate reflection of the practice. *Iso* means "equal," whereas *homeo* means "like." Nosodes are actually derived from the causative agent of a disease, whereas remedies are derived from substances that produce symptoms in a healthy person similar to a certain disease condition.

> ***Some homeopathic physicians have found that nosodes can actually be used in lieu of vaccinations. This is good news for all those parents who are in a quandary over the immunization issue, aware of the dangers of vaccines, but afraid of the consequences of forgoing them entirely. Given the possible contribution of vaccines to the development of autism, avoidance of these "side effects" is a substantial benefit of nosodes.***

For example, the measles nosode is a dilution of the measles virus, and the MMR nosode is a dilution of the MMR vaccine while a homeopathic remedy often used to alleviate a case of measles is *Apis mellifica*, a dilution of a substance derived from bees. *Apis* is indicated for a skin rash that resembles bee stings in appearance and effect, which measles often does. *Apis* may alleviate symptoms of measles infection, but will not clear the measles vaccine from the body, which the nosode can do. This homeopathic application is a single remedy to treat a transitory condition (measles), which is distinct from constitutional homeopathic treatment to rebalance the individual, as discussed in Dr. Reichenberg-Ullman's work.

It is important to note that a nosode, like other homeopathic remedies, does not actually contain any biochemical trace of the substance from which it is derived (in a nosode, a pathogen such as a virus), but is an energetic imprint of that substance. This is why nosodes do not produce the serious side effects associated with vaccines.

There are two strong areas of application for nosodes in relation to autism, one in prevention of the disorder and the other in treatment.

Nosodes: An Alternative to Vaccines

Some homeopathic physicians have found that nosodes can actually be used in lieu of vaccinations. This is good news for all those parents who are in a quandary over the immunization issue, aware of the dangers of vaccines, but afraid of the consequences of forgoing them entirely. Nosodes can prevent the childhood illnesses parents fear, while avoiding the side effects of vaccines. Given the possible contribution of vaccines to the development of autism, avoidance of these "side effects" is a substantial benefit of nosodes.

Richard E. Hiltner, M.D., a family practice physician for 31 years, has not given an immunization shot to a child since 1975. He stopped giving them when he saw first-hand what vaccinations can do. A child he knew was given the standard DPT shot by another doctor. Soon after, the child became mentally retarded and suffered from chronic seizures. The child grew into adulthood with no change in his condition. Witnessing this tragedy was one of the reasons Dr. Hiltner began to study homeopathy.

At the time, he was already searching for another approach to medicine, and this event served as a catalyst for him to make the change. Homeopathy's orientation of treating the whole person, rather than the parts or symptoms, appealed to him particularly. Dr. Hiltner has now been using homeopathy in his practice for 27 years.

Since 1986, he has conducted an informal clinical study. In the normal course of his practice in Ojai, California, he has given approximately 200 children homeopathic nosodes in place of standard immunizations. He follows a typical immunization schedule, using the nosodes for DPT, MMR, and other illnesses for which parents request protection. The outcome of his study reveals that none of the 200 children had problems with the illnesses and none experienced any negative effects from the nosodes.

"I feel that homeopathic immunization nosodes do appear to have some effectiveness in lessening or mitigating the illnesses and therefore should be considered as an alternative to regular immunizations," says Dr. Hiltner. "For those who don't feel comfortable doing nothing [no immunizations] and for those who don't feel comfortable doing the shots, this is a nice happy medium." Dr. Hiltner himself prefers this middle ground as the medical route to take.

Isaac Golden, Ph.D., Di.Hom., N.D., a well-known Australian homeopath and author of *Vaccination? A Review of Risks and Alternatives*, has used nosodes prophylactically with more than 1,000 children. He writes, "[W]hile homoeopathic remedies have been used as safe and effective prophylactics for 200 years, attacks on homoeopathy by some advocates of pharmaceutical medicine have left some parents unsure as to the effectiveness of the homoeopathic alternative."

To address this concern, Dr. Golden conducted a survey of the parents of his young patients who received homeopathic alternatives to vaccines from 1988 to 1993, with a final count of 658 respondents. The results "suggest an efficacy equivalent to conventional vaccines, without serious potential or actual side-effects," he writes in his conclusion to the study.[162]

A colleague of Dr. Hiltner's, Dr. Francisco X. Eizayaga, M.D., a homeopathic physician from Argentina, cites epidemics in history in which homeopathic remedies are recorded to have exerted a strong protective effect. Notably, these have included *Belladonna* during a scarlet fever epidemic in Germany in 1801; *Lathyrus* during a polio epidemic in 1957 in Argentina; the smallpox nosode during a smallpox epidemic in Iowa in 1902; and the meningitis nosode during a meningitis epidemic in Brazil in 1974.

Dr. Eizayaga explains the preventive mechanism: "In homeopathy, we may fulfill a job similar to the one achieved by the vaccines, without any of the inconveniences, with the nosode of each of the acute diseases. While the unspecific resistance of an individual to an infection is increased with the homeopathic remedy, a higher specific immunity against a given germ is obtained with the nosode; in other words, we have certain proofs of specific antibodies being created."[163]

In his clinical practice, Dr. Eizayaga has been using nosodes for many years with great success, both in place of vaccines for childhood illnesses and to prevent the flu. He annually immunizes his patients under 12 years old with nosodes of influenza, tuberculosis, chicken pox, measles, mumps, rubella, pertussis, diphtheria, tetanus, and meningitis, and any others necessary. The dosage schedule is two doses of one nosode only on three consecutive days, with a week in between one nosode and another. If there is an epidemic of a particular illness, he repeats the dosage with the nosode in question. In his many years of following this protocol, he has "observed a very high immunization level" among his patients.

"[I]t would be ideal for our public health authorities to give us the opportunity of showing medical science and public opinion the advantages of an effective, simple, innocuous, and economic homeopathic immunization program," Dr. Eizayaga says.[164]

An excellent source of information about homeopathy and vaccines is the website of Dr. Tinus Smits, a Dutch homeopath who is an authority on vaccines. See www.tinussmits.com.

Nosodes: *Clearing Vaccines*

Nosodes can be highly effective in clearing adverse reactions to vaccines and eliminating or reducing the symptoms of autism related to immunization. In some cases, most of a child's symptoms are the product of this relationship and are resolved upon clearing the energy taint or residue of the toxin from the body. The mechanism by which a nosode clears the vaccine from the body is not entirely understood, just as it is not fully understood exactly how homeopathic remedies work to restore balance in the whole person. The effectiveness of nosodes is clearly demonstrated by clinical results, as discussed in case studies throughout this book.

Carola M. Lage-Roy, a German homeopath (Heilpraktikerin Homoeopathie is the German credential she holds) who also practices in Encinitas, California, has had extensive experience in using nosodes to clear vaccines. She has seen a wide range of problems linked to vaccine damage—not only autism, but also epileptic seizures, brain damage, and paralysis. She has treated quite a few children with autism and seen their symptoms improve or reverse completely after clearing them of the vaccines involved. She notes that more severe cases take longer and often require numerous remedies in addition to nosodes. For example, you can build up the immune system and treat corollary illnesses with homeopathy. The following case history from her files demonstrates the efficacy of nosodes even with long-term autism.

Friedrich: A Teenager with Autism

Friedrich, 16, had been diagnosed with autism around the age of two. He was healthy as a baby and could walk at 11 months. Three days after he got his third DPT vaccination at nine months, he developed a severe case of sinusitis and had to go to the clinic for several days. "This was already vaccine damage," states Lage-Roy.

Immediately following his fourth DPT vaccination at a year and a half, Friedrich became apathetic and withdrawn, and would jump when somebody spoke to him. He had already started talking at that point, but after the shot he stopped. Not long after, he was diagnosed with autism, but no one made any connection between the vaccine and the disorder. Three to four years later, he did slowly begin to speak again, without any intervention, Lage-Roy notes, attributing it to the fact that his family was with him all the time and encouraging him to speak.

Friedrich's father consulted Lage-Roy when his son was sixteen. He had just read one of her books, the *Homeopathic Guide to Vaccine Damages and Treatment*, which suddenly made evident to him that his son's autism was the result of vaccine damage. On his initial visit, Friedrich ran up and down in the clinic, couldn't sit still, and shouted and cried. His father informed Lage-Roy that Friedrich was in a calm period. This behavior was mild compared to what he was like in one of his loud phases, when he was far noisier, became aggressive, and even violent. At other times, he was quiet and withdrawn.

Friedrich, seeing candy on Lage-Roy's desk, repeated the same sentence over and over in an emotionless monotone to her: "He wants a bonbon. He wants a bonbon." In this, he showed the autistic tendency to speak flatly and to refer to oneself in the third person.

Friedrich lived with the family, but it was difficult for them. Every change in the house made him crazy. They bought new doors for the rooms, and he destroyed them all. He also destroyed the toys of his brothers and sisters. The other members of the family had to keep the doors to their rooms closed to protect their belongings. The door to the pantry, particularly, had to be kept closed because he would eat huge amounts of food if he had access. Once, he got in there and ate a whole loaf of bread.

From an early age, Friedrich would run away from home, crying and shouting. The problem was solved when the family got a dog who became attached to Friedrich, took care of him, and wouldn't let him run away.

His father reported that Friedrich didn't like to be touched except to have his father hold his thumbs, which calmed him down. It is interesting to note that in the map of the body in hand reflexology, the thumb corresponds to the brain, so pressing on the thumb would exert healing effects on that area. In addition to the dislike of touch, another of Friedrich's characteristically autistic symptoms was his penchant for smelling everything, particularly new things. He also engaged in repetitive behaviors, for example, sitting for an hour breaking pieces of grass and smelling them, all with no display of affect. Before the onset of the autism, he painted and showed some artistic ability. Afterward, he could only paint a circle with a black point inside it.

In hearing Friedrich's history, Lage-Roy felt that it was obvious that the DPT vaccine was the one implicated in his condition. In her clinical experience with vaccine-induced autism, the problematic vaccine in the DPT triad has been pertussis (whooping cough), as evidenced by the fact that the Pertussis nosode is the one that produces positive changes in the child.

To treat Friedrich, Lage-Roy gave him the Pertussis nosode at a high potency, LM30, which is a high dilution not commonly used in North America. LM remedies are far more dilute (LM means a dilution of 50,000 times) and therefore far more potent than the remedies most homeopaths employ. Lage-Roy has been using these remedies, LM30 and higher, for 20 years in her practice. Despite their potency, the LM remedies are very gentle. She instructs patients to stop taking the remedy in the event they have any uncomfortable reaction. The advantage of these remedies is that any reactions cease very quickly after one discontinues taking them. With the regular high potencies, such as 1M, the reaction can last quite a while after stopping.

A typical dosage Lage-Roy uses to clear vaccines is one dose of the LM30 nosode, taken daily initially, then slowing it down to every fourth day. She asks patients to call her in one to two weeks so she can make sure the remedy is correct for that particular child. At the two-week (maximum) follow-up call, it is normal for the parent to report significant changes, and Lage-Roy can then usually tell if the remedy is working or not.

Friedrich lived in Austria, while Lage-Roy at that time had her practice in Bavaria in Germany. Friedrich's father did not make the follow-up call to Lage-Roy for three months, when he called just to tell her that everything was fine. Friedrich was no longer aggressive or destructive, had joined the family again, and was talking more.

He reported that his son had reacted intensely to the remedy for the first six weeks, with worsening of his behavior. The parents, however, had grown so used to terrible outbursts that for them it was not so abnormal. Lage-Roy learned that Friedrich's father had misunderstood her instructions and had given a dose of the remedy to Friedrich every day until the bottle was empty (about two months). While he was actually going through a very dramatic healing crisis, says Lage-Roy, it wasn't that different from what his life was like anyway. As with his parents, this was, in a sense, normal for Friedrich. "His whole life was a crisis," she notes.

After six weeks, Friedrich suddenly started to remember things that had happened ten years before. He began to speak much more, and related to his parents what he was remembering. He started helping in the household without being asked, which was astonishing to his parents. Before, it had been impossible to get him to do even a little bit in the house.

Lage-Roy relates this case, partly to illustrate how safe homeopathy is, even at the very high potencies. She does not recommend that patients do what Friedrich's father did, however, because it intensifies the healing work of the remedy and can be a heavy experience. Hahnemann's approach with homeopathy was to heal as gently as possible, she notes. But by taking the fast-track approach to healing, Friedrich moved through all the stages rapidly. "After six weeks, he was well on the road to recovery and, in the eyes of his parents, the result was very satisfactory," she says. Normally, when such healing reactions take place, the dose is modified to make the healing process gentler. "But we have observed in other healing cases that heavy reactions are sometimes necessary and so are appropriate."

Lage-Roy called the family a year later because she was curious to know how Friedrich was doing. His father told her that Friedrich still wasn't attending school, but he was talking more and more. His aggression had disappeared; all the doors in the house could be open now. He was helping his mother. "He is fine," concluded the father. "He is making progress, he is helping." The family was happy with that.

The only remedy he received was the pertussis nosode. Lage-Roy would rather have continued to treat Friedrich to effect further progress, but the family was satisfied with what had been achieved. Regarding the autism produced by the vaccination, she notes that it had been effectively reversed by the nosode, as his development restarted after that and progressed continuously. "But more can be done in such cases," says Lage-Roy.

It is sad, she adds, that parents of severely autistic or retarded children are not used to therapeutic intervention producing much change. "For that reason, they are easily satisfied, in my eyes, with small results, and then they stop homeopathic treatment." Knowing what homeopathy can accomplish, it is hard for her to witness this. "I have seen astonishing results with nosodes and all the other homeopathic remedies," she says, citing the following case of a complete reversal of severe vaccine damage.[165]

Multiple Remedies May Be Needed

Lana's parents brought her to Lage-Roy when she was nine months old. A physician had informed them that their child would never walk, that she was just going to lie there her whole life. Not only was she paralyzed, she seemed to be suffering from brain damage, staring stupidly into space. The doctors offered no help to the parents, saying there was no hope. Lana's mother wanted to commit suicide, recalls Lage-Roy.

After Lana's first immunization at three months (she got five vaccines in one), she had begun to exhibit some physical mobility problems. After her six-month shots (again, five at once), her whole body swelled up and she looked as though she had been given cortisone. Unfortunately, the vaccinations were continued according to schedule and with the multiple vaccines. After the nine-month shots, Lana couldn't move at all, not even an arm or a leg. She just lay there and cried.

When Lage-Roy first saw her, Lana's expression was stupid and her eyes vacant. To her astonishment, no one had made the connection between the child's condition and the vaccinations. She treated Lana over the next six years, giving her multiple remedies. She administered the nosodes for all of the vaccines Lana had received. Polio and pertussis were particularly implicated in her case, as demonstrated by the improvements after she took nosodes of those viruses.

Lage-Roy also gave Lana remedies for her symptom picture as it changed. In her practice of homeopathy, she does not use a constitutional remedy according to its normally understood usage, but looks at all the aspects of a person to gain a picture of the patient at that moment in time. "Acute symptoms are especially important in this approach; they are the expression of the deep-seated disease coming up to the surface," she explains.

Lana was often acutely ill and had severe problems with digestion. The latter, along with the paralysis, was an indicator for polio vaccine damage. After Lage-Roy cleared her of the polio vaccine, she was able to sit up. She still didn't react to anything. When people spoke to her, she just stared stupidly at them. Now that she could sit up, she engaged in the repetitious behavior typical of autism, says Lage-Roy.

In the six years that Lage-Roy treated her, Lana received many remedies, as needed with the changes in her condition. Today, she can walk and talk, and is going to school. She laughs now, whereas before she didn't laugh at all. "That was one of the first changes," Lage-Roy recalls. "When she started to get better, she started to laugh."

I include this case, though Lana was physically and mentally disabled in addition to developing autistic symptoms, because it shows an extreme of vaccine damage, which may simply be further along the spectrum from typical autism. Lana's case also illustrates how even extremely severe vaccine damage can be undone to a large extent, which offers hope for parents of children with vaccine-related autism. It will likely require time and multiple homeopathic remedies, but the results support the effort. If vaccines are a factor in a child's autism, at the very least, using nosodes to clear the vaccines seems a wise course to follow. The following case is a sad illustration of how important the monitoring of symptoms is in the homeopathic treatment of autism.

Joseph: The Importance of Monitoring

Joseph was another of Lage-Roy's older autistic patients. His family brought him for treatment when he was 20 years old. His was a very severe case of autism, which also resulted from vaccinations, according to Lage-Roy. It was impossible for the family to have him live with them because he was so aggressive, restless, running around all the time, and generally out of control. He was institutionalized and was receiving twenty-three medication pills a day. Despite the medication, which included Ritalin, he was still aggressive and restless, up in the middle of every night, pounding on the walls when he couldn't sleep.

On one of the holidays when his parents had brought Joseph home, they took him to Lage-Roy to see if she could help. She gave him two nosodes: *Tuberculinum* and *Syphilinum*. He was from Germany, where he had received the tuberculosis vaccination. Given the number of medications he was on, "I thought it was ridiculous to start with just one remedy in this case. I gave him the two remedies together." She also gave him five drops of the two remedies instead of the normal two to three drops because, again, with all the medications, she didn't think the normal dose would have much effect.

In addition, she put the drops in an ounce of water, which potentizes the remedy further, meaning it makes the remedy more powerful. "So five drops of two nosodes in an ounce of water, and this twice a day. This may seem revolutionary to some homeopaths, but common practice to others," she observes. She knew she needed to get fast results because otherwise the family would take him back to the hospital.

The very next day, Joseph was calm. He sat quietly in the kitchen and didn't run around. He was just as calm at night, and his aggression had disappeared. This state of affairs continued for about a week, at which point his old symptoms began to come back. Contrary to Lage-Roy's instructions to call her if there was any change, the parents did not call, and Joseph progressed to his old destructive behavior again as his parents continued to give him the remedy on the prescribed schedule.

Lage-Roy explains that it was clear by the change in his symptom picture that he needed a different remedy to address a new phase he was entering. The parents did finally call Lage-Roy, but only after they had taken their son back to the hospital. After further discussion, however, the family arranged to have Lage-Roy work with Joseph again in the near future, and she believes she can help him.

The lesson of Joseph's story is that parents need to monitor the situation when their child is receiving homeopathic treatment and not just assume that one remedy is going to effect the changes that are needed, even when it initially produces great results. It also highlights the importance of following the homeopath's instructions.

Overall, Lage-Roy's message to parents is: "With homeopathy, there is so much hope for a better and more fruitful life." With less severe cases of autism, she has witnessed reversal numerous times. With severe cases, she has seen great improvement. To date, she has not seen a complete reversal in very severe cases, as treatment needs to be continued over many years.

"I think it's time to stop with any kind of vaccinations," she adds. "They're really not worth the disruption and disease they cause. Childhood illnesses are easy to treat homeopathically. There is no need for vaccinations, and we also have the homeopathic alternatives if people want a safe protection without any side effects."

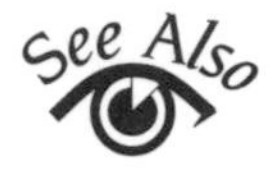

For more about vaccines and autism, see chapters 3 and 8. For more about the use of nosodes in the clearing of vaccines, see chapters 8 and 11.

Treating Childhood Illnesses with Homeopathy

A third area in which homeopathy excels is in the treatment of childhood illnesses. Parents need to know that they have options if they decide to avoid conventional immunizations altogether and/or go the preventive nosode route. In either case, if their child does happen to contract measles, mumps, chicken pox, or other ailment, homeopathic remedies can ease the severity of the illness and shorten its duration.

Many natural medicine practitioners believe that childhood illnesses play an important role in strengthening the immune system, and suppressing these illnesses has deleterious effects on the individual's future health. Philip Incao, M.D., director of a holistic medicine center in Denver, Colorado, is one of these practitioners.[166] He has eschewed the use of most vaccinations in his practice for more than 20 years. "[W]e regard childhood vaccinations as anything but routine; rather, we consider them in most cases to be suspect, dangerous, and worthy of exceedingly rigorous review. Generally, we try to avoid giving most vaccinations and rely instead on alternative, more natural ways of helping the child cope with what we contend are the *necessary* and *beneficial* illnesses of childhood," he says.[167]

You might liken the action of these illnesses to the tempering of steel by fire, the result of which is to leave the metal stronger. In this case, the steel is the immune system. It is not only strengthened in the process, but the fire (the illness) actually contributes to its development. To understand this, we need to consider the two aspects of the immune systems: the humoral immune response and the cell-mediated immune response.

The first involves the production of antibodies (defense proteins) in the blood in response to the presence of foreign antigens (protein markers); immunity or hypersensitivity can result from this reponse. The second involves the production of important immune "workers" (T cells) that migrate around the body, capture microorganisms and antigens, and destroy them or drive them out of the body (through rashes or pus/mucus discharge, which are signs of acute inflammation).

The two aspects of immunity exist in relationship to each other. When the humoral response is overstimulated (by vaccines or allergies, for example), the cell-mediated response becomes less active. Since the latter is the clean-up crew, the contents of vaccines do not get driven out of the body because vaccines do not stimulate cell-mediated activity.

Dr. Inaco defines standard childhood illnesses as acute inflammatory illnesses, typically characterized by fever and rashes. (He does not include polio and tetanus in this category.) He regards them as a developmental phase of childhood. If they are obviated by vaccines, the child misses an important stage in development.

Here's how it works. Vaccines activate the humoral system, while illnesses such as measles, mumps, rubella, chicken pox, or whooping cough develop the cell-mediated system, which must respond to the acute inflammatory state produced by these illnesses. "The difference here is crucial," says Dr. Incao, "because it is the cell-mediated response that protects a child from future illness and that provides, in effect, the deeper immunity."[168]

According to this view, the result of allowing the development of the deeper immunity in childhood is protection against the development of chronic, long-term illnesses in adulthood. Preventing children from contracting these immune-strengthening illnesses can result in a higher incidence of health problems in later life.

Scientists have connected the increasing rates of asthma with the suppression of childhood illnesses, notably those that affect the lungs.[169]

In the case of measles, the virus is normally excreted through the skin via the rash and "burned up" by the fever. With a vaccine, no such clearing takes place because the rash is avoided and the vaccine stimulates the humoral system at the expense of the cell-mediated response. Remaining in the body, the measles virus may chronically irritate the immune system and contribute to the development of degenerative disease, says Dr. Incao.

In an article published in 1985 in *Lancet*, Danish physician Tove Ronne cited the diseases that may develop later in life as a result of measles virus infection without the rash. These included immune dysfunctions, skin disease, degenerative diseases of bone and cartilage, and some cancers.[170] The measles vaccine has also been linked to a higher incidence of inflammatory bowel disease.[171]

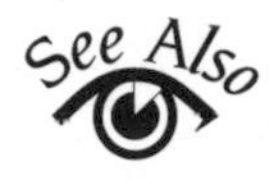

For more about the effects of vaccines, see chapter 3. For more about vaccines and the two aspects of immunity, see chapter 11.

Dr. Incao's approach is to treat the childhood illnesses as they occur with homeopathic or other natural medicines that assist the body in discharging the virus. "The aim of treatment is to support the externalizing and discharging of the illness process—to get it out of the body—so that no residual illness remains to become a chronic problem later in life."[172]

As is true of constitutional homeopathy, the diagnosis (measles, for example) does not determine the remedies that will likely be effective for a given child.

Rather, it is the symptom picture, or the particular manifestations of the illness, in *that* child that indicates the remedies to use. There is no one homeopathic remedy for measles, but many that address the various symptoms. Thus, two children with measles may be taking completely different remedies.

Dr. Incao may use one or a combination of remedies, depending on the child. Homeopathic treatment of acute conditions does not restrict itself to administration of a single remedy. For example, he might give *Apis* to address the bee-sting-like rash of a child's measles, and *Belladonna* to ease the fever. It is important to note that homeopathic remedies, unlike Tylenol, do not suppress the fever, "but allow the constitution to tolerate it better," says Dr. Incao. He reiterates that fever is an essential process for immune health. With homeopathic support, the child can reap the benefits without undue suffering. "The child must be closely observed by a medical professional during the illness process to be sure the course the illness is taking is benign," notes Dr. Incao.[173] This, again, points to the need for parental monitoring of symptoms, so the homeopathic physician can address changes with the appropriate remedy.

In his practice, Dr. Incao has found that about 90 percent of the childhood illnesses in his patients (both the standard ones listed previously and colds, flu, and upper respiratory tract infections conventionally treated with antibiotics) can be eased with about twelve basic low-potency remedies that parents can use at home. He notes that with natural medicine he has also been able for the last 20 years to avoid using antiobiotics to treat children in his practice.[174]

"One of the best ways to ensure your children's health is to allow them to get sick," he summarizes. "The more you allow children to work out their acute illnesses, to really exercise their immune systems without suppressing the process, the stronger the system will be and the less prone the children will be to serious adult degenerative illnesses."[175]

8 *Cranial Osteopathy*: The Role of Birth *Trauma in* Autism

"If we wanted to stop this autism epidemic, we could stop it today. This does not mean cure all autism no matter what the etiology, but definitely stop the epidemic." These are the words of Lawrence Lavine, D.O., M.P.H., D.T.M.&H., whose medical roots are in neurology, neuroepidemiology, and cranial osteopathy. This statement is not high drama to him, but a reasoned assessment based on his clinical observation and research of autism.

According to Dr. Lavine, the epidemic could essentially be over if three practices were instituted: (1) eliminate the at-birth hepatitis B vaccine; (2) give the other standard vaccinations one at a time only (no multiple vaccines) and give them later ("elimination of mercury goes without saying"); and (3) change current standard childbirth practices.

"The epidemic appears to have begun with MMR and accelerated with hepatitis B," states Dr. Lavine, who practices in Tacoma, Washington. "There seems to be a synergistic effect between the two. Additionally, there is a third antecedent factor, and that is the cranial distortions that can be caused by the administration of an epidural and the drug Pitocin." An epidural block, or epidural for short, is a local anesthetic injected into the space around the lower spinal cord for pain relief during childbirth. Pitocin is the drug given to speed the contractions of labor and hurry the process along. The use of both is common in current obstetrical practice.

What Is Cranial Osteopathy?

Cranial osteopathy, developed by William G. Sutherland, D.O., is based on an anatomical and physiological understanding of the interrelationship between mechanisms in the skull (cranium) and the entire body.[176]

The central component of this relationship is what Dr. Sutherland termed the *primary respiratory mechanism*, or PRM. This is "a palpable movement within the body that occurs in conjunction with the motion of the bones of the head."[177]

The cranial bones move rhythmically, alternating between expansion and contraction, and this motion is reflected in every cell of the body. Palpable means that the PRM can be felt anywhere in a patient's body by someone who is trained to feel it; i.e., a person trained in cranial osteopathy. The PRM can be thought of as the intrinsic fluid drive in the system.

As treatment consists of restoring the full functioning of the PRM in the context of the whole body, it is not restricted to the sacrum, spinal cord, and cranium. Cranial osteopaths use gentle, hands-on manipulation and pressure to release areas of restricted motion.

In addition to structural or pain problems, cranial osteopathy can be beneficial for conditions in virtually any system or area of the body, including birth trauma, developmental problems, colic, chronic ear infection, learning disorders, behavior problems, ADD/ADHD, seizures, allergies, asthma, frequent colds or sore throats, and irritable bowel syndrome, among many others.[178]

Cranial osteopathy is not the same as CranioSacral therapy and the terms should not be used interchangeably. For information about CranioSacral therapy, see chapter 9.

What Happens During Birth

While they may be convenient for those involved, these substances can result in the baby's skull being subjected to incredible non-physiologic pressures during birth. As Dr. Lavine explains it, under normal conditions, the woman's pelvis reshapes itself to accommodate birth. This process begins long before the first labor contraction. When the baby drops in late pregnancy, that's already part of the pelvic reshaping.

The reshaping is not a passive process, but an active one involving continual communication via nerve messages passing back and forth between the pelvis, sacral plexus (a network of nerves in the pelvic region/area of the sacrum [lower portion of the spine]), and brain, traveling up and down the spinal cord, and ultimately producing a pituitary hormonal reaction and necessary hormonal secretions. Under normal conditions, the head drops into the pelvis. "The head reshapes and the pelvis reshapes in a kind of 'dance' creating a balance between the head molding and the pelvic molding," says Dr. Lavine. This reshaping continues throughout labor.

If you anesthetize the pelvis, as with an epidural injection, the reshaping that normally occurs is inhibited. When labor does not progress because the vital pelvic involvement has been turned off, Pitocin is introduced to force the uterus to contract artificially. Then, says Dr. Lavine, "It is as though we are using the child's head as a battering ram to force the pelvis to reshape to accommodate it."

Dr. Lavine describes what happens to the infant under these circumstances:

> "When the head comes through the canal, it's pretty liquid. It's like dough, very malleable, very easy to shape. When it comes through, it takes on the form of the maternal pelvis. If you ram the head, you can end up locking a distortion into the head. Typically, when the head comes through, it has to rotate, to twist to get through. What happens [without the normal pelvic reshaping] is you twist and lock. Normally in labor, the head comes through, compresses, twists, then extends, and everything opens up. The mother puts the baby to her breast to nurse, the baby's head pumps itself loose [by the sucking motion], and you've got an internally free-floating head, just the way it's supposed to be. When Pitocin and/or an epidural are used, distortions tend to be locked in."

More About a Baby's Head

A newborn's head is made up of cartilage and membrane, except for two small areas of bone at the lower back of the head (occipital condyle). The cranium is not bone yet because the sections of the skull have to be able to overlap for the head to get through the birth canal. There are two fontanels, or openings, in the membranous areas: the anterior fontanel in the front and the posterior fontanel in the back. These openings and the malleable quality of cartilage and membrane allow for cranial molding as the infant moves through the birth canal, explains Dr. Lavine.

Normally, after the baby has passed through the canal, the fontanels open up. "Especially if you put the baby to the breast," says Dr. Lavine. "The force of sucking on the breast tissue puts force and stress, hydraulic pressure, up through the top of the mouth, and transmits the force into the cranial base. That opens up the whole head, which allows for normal cranial dynamics to take place."

The fontanels are there for the labor process and don't seem to serve much purpose after birth. "But if they're closed immediately after delivery, it tells you that things are not working correctly," says Dr. Lavine. Closed fontanels indicate a misalignment of the cranial base, which is the base of the entire skull, where all the structures of the skull attach. If the cranial base is out of alignment, nothing that attaches to it can be in alignment.

A head misshapen by a traumatic birth is not able to function optimally, he says, contrary to the more common view that it is not a matter of concern and the child will grow out of it. In addition to the direct effects of compression on the brain, there are compressions of cranial nerves as well as systemic effects resulting from disturbance in the primary respiratory mechanism (see sidebar, "What Is Cranial Osteopathy?") of the body, the proper function of which depends upon the free contraction and expansion of the cranium.

When an epidural and Pitocin are required due to some obstetrical process, then the newborn would benefit immensely from cranial osteopathic treatment as soon as possible after delivery, says Dr. Lavine.

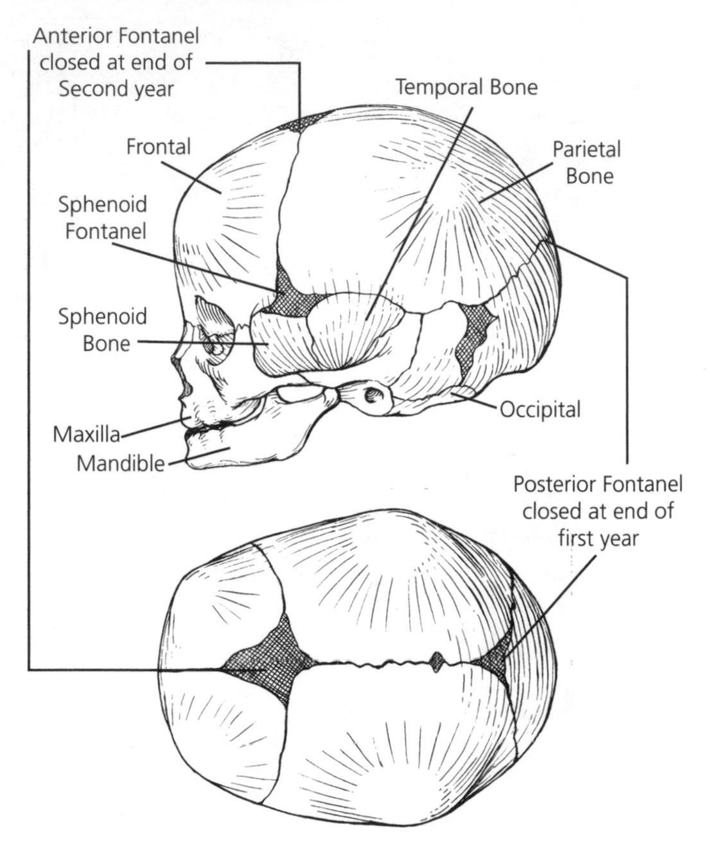

Fontanels of Infant's Skull and the Main Bones of Skull

Here we arrive at information that may help explain a piece of the mystery surrounding autism. We have already learned of the extent to which biochemistry plays a role in this condition still categorized by some as a psychiatric disorder. Now, we are presented with a purely structural component. A specific type of compression (of the left middle cranial fossa; explanation follows) and locking is often seen in children diagnosed with autism. Other, more common types of compression and cranial distortion are seen in cases of ADD or ADHD.

That the development of these disorders is potentially greater when vaccines are given on top of the cranial irritation that results from the distortions and locks is of great concern to Dr. Lavine. Clearly, not all infants who suffer from this compression of the left middle cranial fossa during birth will develop autism, but the majority of children he has studied who do develop autism evidence this compression pattern, as can be seen in osteopathic examination and MRIs (magnetic resonance imaging, a scanning technique based on electromagnetic energy rather than the radiation used in X rays).

To test what he observed through years of osteopathic practice, Dr. Lavine reviewed the charts of twenty-five children who were consecutively brought to him for treatment and who fit the diagnostic category of autistic disorder as defined by the *DSM-IV*. He found that twenty-two of the twenty-five children had compression of the left middle cranial fossa, among other shared distortions.[179] This trend appears in MRIs of autistic children; Dr. Lavine notes that it was in looking at an MRI in a paper published by Dr. Eric Courchene from San Diego that brought this trend into focus for him.[180]

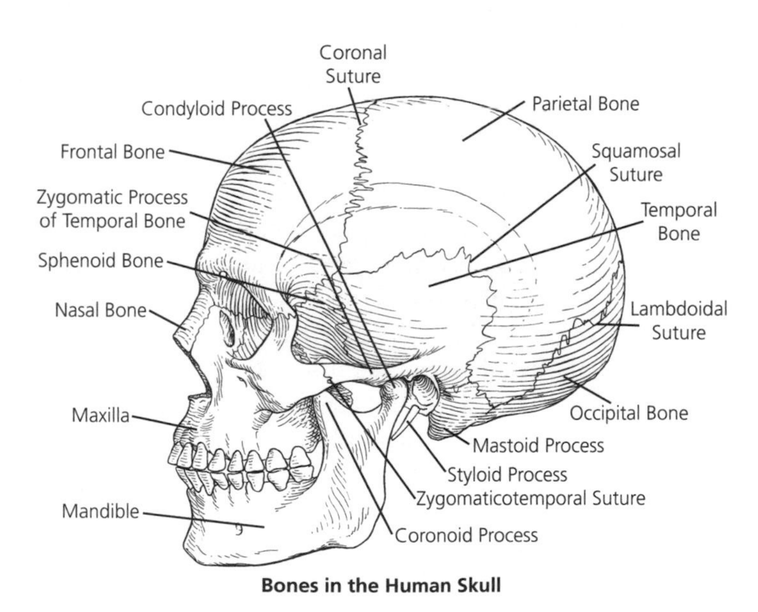

Bones in the Human Skull

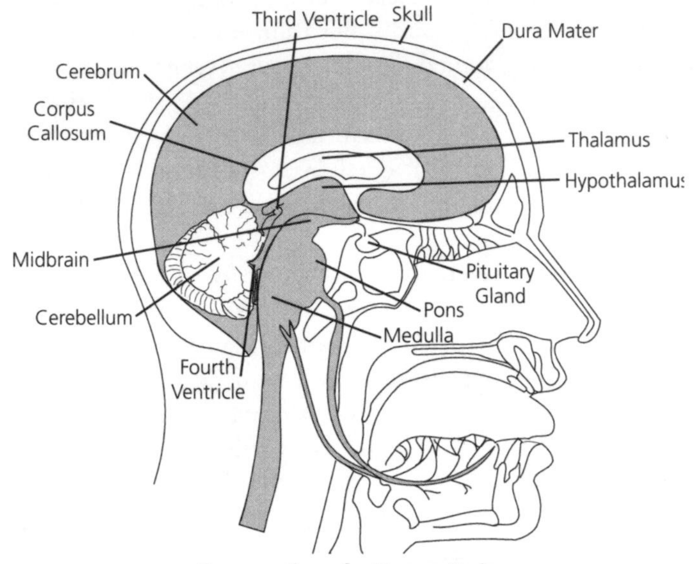

Cross-section of a Human Brain

What are the structural and developmental effects on the body of this twist and the other birth-induced cranial distortions? Dr. Lavine explains:

"With the compressions and locks, several things can happen. With autism, you wind up in primarily a flexion pattern. Flexion is defined osteopathically as when the sphenobasilar symphysis ascends. What this means is that the joint formed by the occiput and the sphenoid (a large bat-wing-shaped bone deep inside the head) lifts up; it is then said to be 'in flexion.' When this distortion is created, the falx (the big, thick band of tissue on top of the head that runs from front to back) gets pulled down tight, putting pressure on the corpus callosum, the thick area or band of brain tissue that connects one hemisphere to the other. The result of that is compromised communication from one side of the brain to the other.

"Additionally, the tentorium [the tentlike structure between the cerebrum and the cerebellum] is pulled down flat, resulting in compression on the cerebellum, the area of the brain that contributes to socialization, motor planning, motor movement, etc.

"Due to the complex restrictions, compression occurs in the left middle cranial fossa. In the cranium, there are three pairs of pans or depressions. The frontal lobe [of the brain, with right and left hemispheres] sits in the front pan, or fossa. The temporal lobe or speech center sits in the middle pan. The cerebellum sits in the back pan.

"At age 15 to 18 months, when speech starts to develop, there is tremendous growth in the middle cranial fossa. If there haven't been any external assaults, such as multiple vaccines given in close temporal proximity on [top of] an already low-grade brain irritability caused by the birth process, the brain can tolerate this compression because the vault responds to maintain a normal balance of brain to surrounding membranes. (Remember, the bones/cartilage sit inside of a membranous sack and change shape in response to the pressure and stress from those membranes.)

"Speech may be delayed, or some speech problems may be evident, but the child can do well. Often you wouldn't even know there's a problem. But when you put any other type of stress on top of the compression, the scene is at least set for potential problems."

The cranial strain pattern makes the brain irritable, and this irritability makes the brain far more vulnerable to adverse environmental influences such as vaccines, mercury, and other toxins.[181]

Age 15 to 18 months is when children get the MMR vaccination. So, just at the time when they are experiencing maximum cranial growth and development, especially in the speech areas, they are given a vaccine, which is a potential trauma and a potential poison to the system. All of the components of the vaccine are foreign substances and can potentially cause problems, says Dr. Lavine. "The vaccine often causes a low-grade encephalitis, an actual brain irritation."

Under the influence of the combination of the left middle cranial fossa compression on the speech centers and low-grade brain irritability, these children stop talking, are no longer developmentally in synch with their peers, and may even regress. Dr. Lavine notes that if the child has not had the hepatitis B vaccination, the problems may be less severe, but MMR alone can push a predisposed system toward autism when combined with the cranial distortions.

Autism, in most cases, is a multifactorial condition, says Dr. Lavine. "The system under any given circumstance has a tremendous amount of resiliency. But if you push it too far, it decompensates or goes out of balance, and when that happens any number of disorders can present."

The compression of the infant's head can also be caused by a distortion in the mother's pelvis. As noted before, during birth the baby's head molds to the shape of her pelvis. Cranial osteopathy can correct the mother's pelvic distortion before or even during labor, allowing the child to be born with a normal-shaped head, provided that an epidural and Pitocin are not used, since they can interfere with the process.

Dr. Lavine is not suggesting that women go through labor in agonizing pain. He is advocating the reclamation of natural practices that reduce the pain, such as the methods long known to midwives and osteopaths for assisting the pelvis in reshaping itself to accommodate the passage of the baby through the birth canal. Laboring in a hot water bath can also reduce the pain of contractions. "The labor pain can drop dramatically," notes Dr. Lavine. "Most women can handle the pain that remains without too much trouble." If an epidural and Pitocin are used, he urges parents to get osteopathic treatment for their infant immediately after birth, while the head is still liquid (easy to reshape).

Many parents have brought their babies to Dr. Lavine in the month or so after birth because they are concerned about the misshapen head. They have often been told by other doctors that the child will grow out of it. "Typically, they are not going to grow out of it," says Dr. Lavine, and given the previous discussion, it may be essential to correct the problem. Cranial osteopathy releases the locked state of the baby's skull and restores it to its natural fluidity. In the process, the soft spot (the anterior fontanel) that wasn't there reopens. As stated in the sidebar, "More About a Baby's Head," when the fontanel is closed after delivery, it is an indication of a misalignment.

As with the other therapies discussed in this book, the earlier the intervention can take place, the better. However, cranial osteopathy can be implemented at any age, says Dr. Lavine. What is specifically accomplished therapeutically, he explains, is to get the child out of the locked flexion; to get the falx to release, thus taking the pressure off the connection between the two hemispheres; to get the pressure off the back of the brain so the socialization and motor functions of the cerebellum are free to develop; and to remove the compression in the left middle cranial fossa and thus take the pressure off the speech centers of the temporal lobe. All of this gives the brain the room to start to grow as it needs to for the proper development of all functions.

If cranial osteopathy was not done at birth and the child's development has been delayed by the compression on the brain, then some kind of intensive rehabilitation, such as speech therapy, occupational therapy, physical therapy, and/or sensory integration therapy, will be necessary, according to Dr. Lavine. "The idea is to turn those functions back on and get them back on track developmentally."

Family Experience

It was through a family member that Dr. Lavine made the connection among cranial distortions, vaccines, and autism. In 1994, after receiving the MMR at 15 months of age, Dr. Lavine's young relative stopped talking. Upon receiving the diagnosis of autism, the parents asked the specialty team, "What do we do?" The response was "There is nothing we can really tell you that works; call the Autism Society." That's the typical answer most parents got then, Dr. Lavine says. "Unfortunately, many parents are still not being made aware of the many therapies available. While there is no 'silver bullet,' and not every intervention will be effective with every child, there are now many more treatment options."

At that point, Dr. Lavine began to research the disorder. "I sat down, and in two weeks read seven hundred pages of journal articles, a flood of abstracts, and several books, and talked to numerous specialists." By then, Dr. Lavine had been practicing cranial osteopathy for 20 years, although not on a full-time basis. He knew the significance of the cranial distortions that could happen at birth. Following the diagnosis of autism, the little boy had several sessions of osteopathic treatment. One weekend, after two treatments on two consecutive days, "we had direct eye contact for the first time in a year," recalls Dr. Lavine. "It was that dramatic."

Recovery was under way, but full recovery takes time, he cautions. "In my relative's case, it took two and a half years to bring him to a normal age functioning level." In addition to cranial osteopathy, other treament modalities used were homeopathy, allergy elimination (NAET), nutritional supplements, and intensive rehabilitation with speech therapy, Applied Behavior Analysis (ABA), auditory integration therapy, sensory integration therapy, and specialized computer programs. Now nine, the boy is functioning at a normal level developmentally, academically, and socially.

His experience with his relative's disorder precipitated a change in Dr. Lavine's clinical practice. In 1996, he made the shift from allopathic medicine to a practice focused on osteopathic manipulative medicine, homeopathy, and other forms of complementary and alternative medicine. Autism is one of his primary clinical foci, and to date he has treated more than fifty children with the disorder.

Components of Treatment

Through his experience with autistic children, Dr. Lavine has found that a combination of therapeutic interventions works best in the treatment of autism. The components he provides are: cranial osteopathic treatment, the elimination of allergies with NAET (Nambudripad's Allergy Elimination Techniques), and the clearing of vaccine reactions with isopathy (homeopathic nosodes). Other therapies (delivered by multiple practitioners) Dr. Lavine cites as often critical to a child's total treatment program are: correcting digestion and the lipid metabolism problem so common to autistic children; nutrient supplementation; heavy metal detoxification; and ABA, speech therapy, sensory integration therapy, auditory integration therapy, and/or other rehabilitative interventions needed by an individual child.

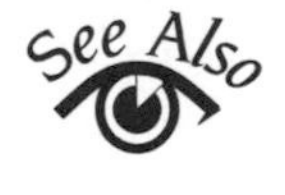

For more about NAET, see chapter 5; for isopathy (nosodes), see chapter 7; for digestive/nutritional therapy, see chapter 4; and for a sensory integration therapy, see chapter 10.

In Dr. Lavine's study of the twenty-five children discussed earlier, the combination of some or all of the previously mentioned treatments produced the following outcomes: fifteen of the twenty-five children now talk in sentences of four or more words, initiate social interaction, and engage in imaginative play; and regarding school, one of the twenty-five is fully recovered and attending a regular classroom, eleven attend a regular classroom with some special assistance, and the other thirteen are in special school programs for autistic children.

Dr. Lavine has found that a combination of therapeutic interventions works best in the treatment of autism. The components he provides are: cranial osteopathic treatment, the elimination of allergies with NAET, and the clearing of vaccine reactions with isopathy (homeopathic nosodes).

Again, Dr. Lavine emphasizes that "no 'magic bullet,' no single treatment alone, was found to significantly ameliorate or reverse the effects of autism. Instead, in all cases an individualized, well thought out and integrated approach was required to move these children along the road to improvement and recovery."[182]

Dr. Lavine cautions that when one is using natural medicine, it is important to understand what is known as "the healing crisis," a temporary worsening of symptoms (in the case of autism, this would also include behavior) with treatment. The healing crisis usually doesn't last long, and it commonly presages a marked improvement in functioning. Systems of medicine used around the world for thousands of years, such as Ayurvedic medicine and traditional Chinese medicine (TCM), have long addressed the healing crisis. Parents need to be aware of the phenomenon, says Dr. Lavine, so they are prepared for the probability of their child's condition getting slightly worse before getting better.

Allergies and Autism

As previously discussed, the brain of an autistic child can potentially be doubly irritated: first, by the compression on the brain from birth; and second, by vaccines. With the digestive compromise that usually ensues, leaky gut syndrome and its attendant allergies are common. With the toxic effect of substances (food molecules) not normally found in the bloodstream (as in leaky gut) and continual allergic reaction, the brain may then be triply irritated, says Dr. Lavine.

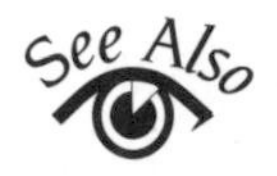

For more about leaky gut syndrome and allergies, see chapter 4.

Further, cranial compression disturbs neurotransmitter function. Many autistic children wind up with allergies to their own neurotransmitters, states Dr. Lavine. "That's one of the reasons Dr. Devi Nambudripad is getting such good results with just NAET." The allergic factor explains the high level of serotonin often present in autistic children. With an allergy to the neurotransmitter, the body doesn't recognize its own serotonin, instead regarding it as a foreign substance. The feedback mechanism sends the message that more serotonin is needed, so the body just keeps producing it, but the brain is unable to utilize it.

Dr. Lavine uses NAET to identify and eliminate the allergies of the children with autism in his practice. Like Dr. Nambudripad, he has discovered that the children show allergies to vaccines they have received. "We're finding that 100 percent of these kids are allergic to the hepatitis B and MMR vaccines," he says. In his experience, an allergy to DPT is also common, but not as prevalent as the other two vaccines. Dr. Lavine observes that the body seems better able to tolerate the polio vaccine, perhaps because it is given orally.

A Word About Vaccines

Dr. Lavine employs homeopathy in four ways in relation to the issue of vaccines: (1) to clear adverse reactions to vaccines; (2) as an alternative to vaccines; (3) to treat illnesses when they arise; and (4) as a constitutional remedy for holistic treatment. The first two involve the use of nosodes (isopathy).

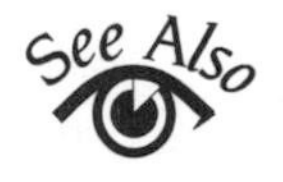

For more about homeopathy and vaccines, see chapter 7.

If the child does contract one of the standard childhood illnesses, Dr. Lavine has found that homeopathic remedies can be very effective in alleviating them. "There are good remedies for many of the childhood diseases." He cites the example of a chickenpox outbreak that occurred in Tacoma about three years ago. Thirteen of the fourteen children with chickenpox in his practice responded positively to the homeopathic remedy *Rhus toxicodendron,* commonly used for the ailment. The fourteenth child did not respond to *Rhus tox,* but did respond to another remedy.

"People get very concerned about serious effects of childhood diseases," observes Dr. Lavine, "but homeopathy can often not only diminish symptoms, but also prevent the illness from becoming serious." In addition, he says, "There is no question that in most cases natural disease, especially if you get the illnesses when you are young, is much less detrimental to the system. The MMR has generated far more disease than measles ever did. This is an issue that needs to be looked at critically and without bias by the scientific and epidemiologic community."

As discussed in chapter 7, the use of nosodes of the various childhood illnesses can sometimes replace vaccination, thus avoiding the potentially deleterious effects and risks of conventional vaccines. Dr. Lavine prefers this approach, but if parents feel more comfortable vaccinating, he, like many other natural medicine practitioners, recommends splitting up the MMR and giving each viral component as a single injection, spaced at least three to four weeks apart, and not administered until the child is nine months old at the earliest. Two or three years old is preferable, he notes.

When parents want a vaccine, Dr. Lavine uses NAET and homeopathy to dramatically reduce and often eliminate side effects and reactions. "If you're really scared to death of measles, then by all means get an individual measles shot," he says. Rubella, the third component of the MMR, is a mild disease. "It is not of real concern except to pregnant women." His suggestion is to vaccinate post-pubertal girls, if they haven't already had rubella as a childhood disease. As for the second component of the triple vaccination, "mumps can theoretically leave people sterile, but not if you get mumps before puberty. You could vaccinate at age four or five," he suggests.

For sources of information on vaccines, their alternatives, and homeopathic approaches, see the recommended reading and list of websites in appendix B.

Children with autism may still suffer the damaging effects of vaccines, even if they have not been immunized, cautions Dr. Lavine. One child in his practice had never been vaccinated. He had the typical cranial distortion, but resolving that problem didn't produce the expected changes in his condition. A blood test revealed vaccine antibodies to several of the childhood vaccines (the test distinguishes between natural and vaccine antibodies). "The vaccines are so ubiquitous, they can be found everywhere," says Dr. Lavine. They have entered our water and food supply because all those who receive the shots excrete the vaccines in their saliva, urine, and stool.

Johnny: The Triple Load

When Johnny's mother brought him to Dr. Lavine, he was three and a half years old and had been diagnosed with autism a

Colic: A Simple Example of What Cranial Compression Can Do

Structurally induced infant colic can usually be resolved in one cranial osteopathic treatment, according to Dr. Lavine. "Cranial osteopaths have been treating babies for 50 to 60 years with predictable, uniform results." One form of colic is caused by compression and the attendant irritation of the tenth cranial nerve (the vagus nerve) due to birth-induced skull distortion, he explains. This nerve supplies all the organs in the abdominal cavity, so it is integral to digestion.

The ninth, tenth, and eleventh cranial nerves come through the jugular foramen (hole), along with the jugular vein, at the base of the skull. The twelfth cranial nerve, the hypoglossal nerve, comes through the hypoglossal canal also at the cranial base. This nerve supplies the muscles of the tongue, and thus is involved in the sucking motion of nursing.

When the base of the skull is out of alignment, compression of the tenth and twelfth nerves can result, producing problems in the areas of the body fed by these nerves. Cranial osteopathic treatment realigns the skull and removes the compression on the nerves. "The colic goes away, the infant starts sucking again, and everyone gets some sleep," says Dr. Lavine.

Parenthetically, he adds that he is seeing with increased frequency another form of colic, and that is colic secondary to an allergy to breast milk. "This particularly seems to occur with mothers who have mercury amalgam fillings in their teeth," he adds. In such cases, he treats the child with NAET to clear the allergy to breast milk and then to mercury. Dr. Lavine concludes, "This mercury amalgam load may also interact with the mercury in vaccines to increase the level of mercury toxicity and overall mercury burden on the central nervous system."

year earlier. After his MMR vaccination, he had regressed; he stopped talking, withdrew from socialization, had periods of wild, out-of-control behavior, and exhibited numerous other characteristically autistic behaviors. Dr. Lavine learned that Johnny's was an epidural-Pitocin delivery, and he had received the hepatitis B vaccine as well as all the other inoculations according to the usual schedule.

It took three cranial osteopathic treatments to resolve the classic twist and compressions of Johnny's skull and fully release its locked state. Dr. Lavine then tested Johnny for allergies and discovered that he was allergic to almost all of the foods/substances in NAET's twelve basic groups. He was also allergic to MMR, hepatitis B, and mercury.

After using NAET to eliminate all of these allergies, Dr. Lavine focused on homeopathic treatment to clear the vaccine reactions from Johnny's body. Many practitioners use muscle response testing (see chapter 5) to determine the most effective homeopathic potency for a particular individual. Dr. Lavine uses cranial osteopathy to read the response of the primary respiratory mechanism (see sidebar, "What Is Cranial Osteopathy?") to proposed potencies.

For this, he puts his hands on the patient's head to monitor the response. He then places on the child's stomach or chest a homeopathic vial containing a 30C potency of a vaccine, and tests an array of vaccines in turn to determine which nosode to use. He then uses an array of that particular nosode to determine the potency needed according to the CRI (cranial rhythmic impulse, or fluid drive). He uses this same method to determine the appropriate order for vaccine clearing. "The body tells us which one it wants treated, and in what order," Dr. Lavine says. He notes that he tests "blind," meaning he doesn't know which vaccine or potency he is testing.

In Johnny's case, each nosode treatment brought "a dramatic improvement," according to Dr. Lavine, who reports that this is quite typical in his experience. The improvements included increased meaningful speech, socialization, and eye contact, and decreased inappropriate behaviors. Behavior seems particularly impacted by the nosodes. "These children tend to be greatly out of sync with their environment in large part because they have pronounced sensory integration issues," says Dr. Lavine. Their typically positive response to the vaccine nosodes can be viewed as indirect support that vaccines are indeed a contributing factor to autism. "You treat the vaccine [presence] homeopathically, and there is improvement. Why would this improvement occur if the child's condition wasn't at least partially caused by the vaccine?"

The response is sometimes direct and immediate; at other times, it is more subtle. The effects of homeopathic nosode treatment tend not to be transitory. Occasionally, retreatment is required, but investigation usually reveals that the homeopathic remedy was antidoted (cancelled out) in some way. In those instances, the dose simply needs to be readministered.

It has now been three years since Johnny first came for treatment. Dr. Lavine reports that he is "incredibly articulate" and is in a regular classroom without an aide. Although Johnny's condition greatly improved following the cranial osteopathy, allergy elimination, and vaccine clearing, his recovery required speech and other rehabilitative therapies. Initially on an intense therapeutic schedule, he is now down to once weekly occupational therapy/speech sessions.

Dr. Lavine has become an adamant proponent of doing whatever is necessary to stop the current epidemic. "The bottom line is prevention. We can stop this. . . . A sensible and reasoned approach to the birth process and vaccinations now can only help speed the end to what has become an epidemic of autism."

Johnny continues to get osteopathic treatment once a month to ensure that cranial relocking doesn't occur. "The cells in the body have an incredible intellect," explains Dr. Lavine. "You have these distortions, and the cells know of the distortions. You have to treat them as the children grow, or they can potentially lock themselves back up again." In addition, the typical falls and bang-ups of childhood can again throw out alignment. For autistic children, who have already been neurologically compromised, it is especially important not to allow any misalignment to persist. Those patients who have recovered to a significant degree see Dr. Lavine only every three to six months, with a visit as needed if there is any significant trauma.

Summing Up

Having seen—in his own family and in his patients—that children can recover from autism, Dr. Lavine has become an adamant proponent of doing whatever is necessary to stop the current epidemic. "The bottom line is prevention. We can stop this. While many investigators are doing valuable research that will come to fruition in time, a sensible and reasoned approach to the birth process and vaccinations now can only help speed the end to what has become an epidemic of autism."

9 Soma Therapies: Structural, Functional, and Emotional Release

Like Dr. Lavine in chapter 8, Zannah Steiner, C.M.P., R.M.T., founder and clinic director of Soma Therapy Centre in Vancouver, British Columbia, has seen numerous cases of autism, ADD/ADHD, and other developmental delays that are linked to structural distortions from birth trauma. She uses the soma (body) therapies CranioSacral therapy, Visceral Manipulation, and SomatoEmotional Release to address these distortions. By combining these methods, the structural, functional, and emotional results of trauma can be released and the just-mentioned conditions significantly ameliorated.

Specifically, CranioSacral therapy corrects the distortions and compressions resulting from birth trauma and restores the previously impeded flow of cerebrospinal fluid (the fluid that bathes the brain and spinal cord). Visceral manipulation restores organ function, which is disturbed by structural interferences, the poor flow of cerebrospinal fluid, and blockages in the flow of energy and nutrients throughout the body.

SomatoEmotional Release assists the body in discharging the stored emotions that result from trauma and that block the body's energy flow, further contributing to physical dysfunction. The body-mind link is clearly evident in the effects of trauma on the body, as one dysfunction contributes to another. For healing to be comprehensive, all of these effects need to be addressed in therapeutic intervention.

Before we turn to the specifics of what Steiner has discovered about autism in her work, it's important to note that she, like many natural medicine practitioners, does not employ the conventional diagnostic label to guide her treatment approach. The only purpose served by the labels with which the children arrive at her clinic may be in the corollary information of how many of those bearing the diagnoses mentioned have similar cranial distortions. This information is important for parents to be aware of, as Dr. Lavine highlighted, and can add to the body of evidence suggesting that cranial osteopathic or CranioSacral measures should be taken immediately after birth to prevent the development of autistic characteristics or other disorders in a child who suffered distortions and compressions during the birth process. Steiner believes that treating newborns with one of these techniques should be routine practice.

Soma Therapies

The following techniques are the primary soma (body) therapies used by Zannah Steiner and her colleagues at Soma Therapy Centre:

CranioSacral therapy (CST) was developed by osteopathic physician John Upledger, who defines CST as "a gentle, hands-on method of evaluating and enhancing the functioning of a physiological body system called the craniosacral system—comprised of the dural membranes and cerebrospinal fluid (CSF) that surround and protect the brain and spinal cord."[183] The word 'craniosacral' derives from the two poles of this system: the sacrum (base of the spine) and the cranium (the skull).

The skull is composed of interlocking bone plates that are far more moveable than most people think. Accident, injury, and the birth process can cause misalignment of the bone plates, resulting in what is termed cranial distortion. This distortion can in turn exert pressure on the brain (compression) and impede the proper flow of CSF. This compression in the skull and impeded CSF flow can produce symptoms throughout the body, from the more obvious such as headaches and back pain to less obvious breathing and digestive disorders.[184]

By releasing restrictions in this system through gentle adjustments, CST improves central nervous system function and has beneficial effects for many health conditions. According to the Upledger Institute, these include motor-coordination impairments, colic, autism, central nervous system disorders, infantile disorders, learning disabilities, immune disorders, chronic fatigue, emotional difficulties, stress and tension-related problems, fibromyalgia and other connective-tissue disorders, temporomandibular joint syndrome (TMJ), post-traumatic stress disorder, orthopedic problems, migraine headaches, and chronic neck and back pain.[185]

Visceral Manipulation, a therapeutic technique for relieving restrictions and tensions in and around organs (viscera), was developed by French osteopath Jean-Pierre Barral in the early 1970s. "The basic philosophy of Visceral Manipulation is that an organ in good health has good movement," Zannah Steiner explains. When tissue becomes rigid or fixed, chronic irritation and dysfunction result. The function of surrounding tissues is also compromised as they attempt to adapt to their altered neighbors.

According to Dr. Barral, each organ in the body has its own biological rhythm, moving through five to eight cycles per minute. It also moves subtly, rotating around what Dr. Barral termed its own "embryogenic axis," which is the orientation it had when the fetal organs were developing. Scar tissue from surgery or injury, chronic inflammation, or shortened fascia (fibrous connective tissue) can disturb the rhythm and rotation of organs. Through specifically applied, light manual force, Visceral Manipulation releases the tensions and restrictions, and restores the proper mobility and inherent rhythm of the organs.

In addition to improved organ function, resulting benefits are better fluid circulation, relief of sphincter and muscle spasms, relief of chronic pain and tension, improved digestion and hormonal balance, and enhancement of localized and systemic immunity. "The organ system can be a storage facility of unexpressed emotion," says Steiner. "The organs are thought to contain the 'voice of the body.'" Thus, Visceral Manipulation can also release emotional holding. With the therapy, patients often experience a sense of well-being.[186]

SomatoEmotional Release (SER), an offshoot of CST, is a hands-on technique developed around 1980 by Dr. Upledger and biophysicist Zvi Karni, Ph.D. The SER works to aid the body in releasing the residual effects of past traumas which can be viral, bacterial, emotional, or physical, as from an injury or structural damage.

A trauma results in the formation of what Dr. Upledger termed "energy cysts" as the body walls off the trauma to store it locally rather than allowing it to become systemic. Just as the body creates inflammation around the puncture site after you step on a nail, it forms an energy cyst in the body to contain the residues of strong emotions such as fear, anger, or resentment, that remain in the body after a traumatic emotional event.

For example, if as a child your mother looked at you with eyes like daggers, your body may have experienced it like a stab to the heart. The body then walled off the energy residues in that area, creating an energy cyst in your chest. Or it could be stored in muscles or organs anywhere in the body. These energy cysts restrict the body's free flow of energy and movement, and may become a localized source of dysfunction and produce discomfort.[187]

Through light touch on areas where energy cysts are located, the SER therapist works with the patient's body-mind to release the emotional content of the blockages, relying on the messages communicated by the craniosacral system as a guide. The release often triggers memory of the event and patients may even assume the position they were in when the injury or trauma occurred.

While some patients engage with the therapist in what is termed in SER "reflective dialogue technique," talking about what they are feeling in the process, the experience need not be articulated. It is as effective on a preverbal or nonverbal level, which makes SER an excellent method for releasing the residues of past traumas in infants and children.

The release of energy cysts often produces immediate emotional and physical benefits. As SER helps restore the free flow and energy and movement in the body, the conditions that can be ameliorated by the therapy may be limitless. Among those that Zannah Steiner cites as responding well are neurological disorders, mental disorders, chronic pain, whiplash, and degenerative diseases.

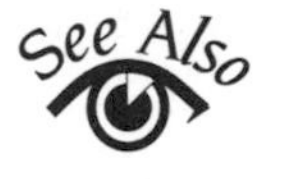

For details on the physiological concepts referred to in this chapter, and more about birth trauma and autism, see chapter 8.

The Nature of Birth Trauma

Steiner distinguishes between "true" autism, which is viewed as a genetic disorder and typically presents with some degree of mental retardation, and autisoid (autistic-like) behaviors caused by environmental factors such as birth trauma. In the latter case, "the birth trauma is presenting itself in the same way as an autistic presentation," she says. In Steiner's clinical experience, the

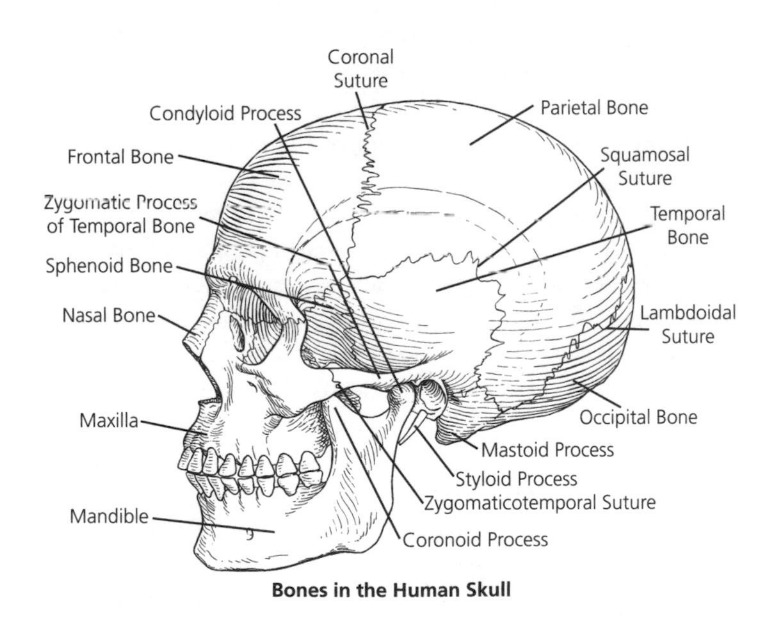

Bones in the Human Skull

coronal suture of children who are autisoid or labeled autistic typically is fixed, or immobile. The coronal suture is the line of union between the parietal and frontal bones of the skull; it runs like a hair band from one ear to the other across the top of the head. When this suture joint is fixed, in its entirety or, more usually, on one side or the other, it restricts the normal movement of the bones of the head, the dural membranes, and cerebrospinal fluid (CSF) flow.

Steiner's analysis of birth-induced distortions is similar to Dr. Lavine's, but she describes the process slightly differently. The suture problem may result from the head being torqued or compacted in the birth canal, or from the baby being stuck there for a prolonged period of time, she says. When the latter happens, the sutures seize up, locking the bones of the skull into an overlapped position; the bones naturally overlap in order for the head to make the passage through the canal.

"When an infant who becomes lodged in the birth canal in this way is then delivered by cesarean section, the cranial bones are much like a flower with its petals folded in on each other," says Steiner. Normally, as the baby's head emerges from the birth canal, the cranial bones that have overlapped to allow passage decompress sequentially, "much like a flower blooming." The first real bathing by cerebrospinal fluid of the brain happens at this point, she adds.

Babies who get stuck and are then removed via C-section miss the sequential compression and decompression of the bones. The "blossoming" may never take place (without therapeutic intervention). Or to use another metaphor, "The baby that's been in the birth canal for a prolonged period, and then is taken by C-section, is like the scuba diver that surfaces too quickly from a subatmospheric pressure to an atmospheric pressure," Steiner says. In the baby's case, the sudden change from the subatmospheric pressure of the womb to the atmospheric pressure of the outside world with its gravitational forces adds additional resistance to CSF flow and further contributes to compression.

As discussed in the previous chapter, the distortions and rigidity in the skull can have far-reaching neurological, behavioral, mental, and functional effects. Autistic or, as Steiner prefers, "autisoid" manifestations may ensue. Fortunately, "when you release the fixed sutures and get the cerebrospinal fluid flowing, results can occur really fast. We can see immediate behavioral, neurological, and functional changes," she says. Parenthetically, Steiner notes that the head-hitting exhibited by many autistic children may be the child's attempt to alleviate or release the constant pressure in the head caused by the cranial distortions.[188]

Let's look at a case from Steiner's patient files to see how CranioSacral therapy, Visceral Manipulation, and SomatoEmotional Release work in treating an autisoid child.

Peter: Structural and Emotional Release

Peter was a healthy baby until 20 months old, at which point he suddenly lost his well-developed vocabulary and subsided into incommunicativeness. His behavior changed dramatically as well. He began to avoid eye contact, seemed overwhelmed by even slight stimulation, and took to banging his head against the wall and hitting himself in the face. When people asked him a question, he screamed or made unintelligible noises. Whereas before he had been a good sleeper, he now slept for only four hours or fewer each night. His previously healthy appetite also changed for the worse and, as time went on, he began to look wan and sickly. His motor coordination regressed, and he could no longer walk without help.

When Peter's mother brought him to Zannah Steiner, she had been trying for two years to get answers to what was wrong with her son. She had finally gotten the diagnosis of autistic spectrum disorder for him, but doctors had no solutions, and Peter had remained about the same, with normal development seemingly on hold.

At Soma Therapy Centre, examination using CST methodology (which includes evaluation of the craniosacral system) revealed restricted cerebrospinal fluid flow. In CST parlance, the craniosacral system, which drives the flow of cerebrospinal fluid, functions as a semi-closed hydraulic pumping mechanism. "That pumping mechanism is responsible for ensuring that all of the fluids of the body are flowing," says Steiner.

"Cerebrospinal fluid is the body's most important fluid. It is the basic soup stock of the body, containing the ingredients—proteins, enzymes, and electrolytes—that are the basis of all other fluid systems." When CSF flow is diminished, fewer nutrients and less oxygen are delivered, and all other fluid systems are compromised. Thus, less CSF means less of everything else.

Without the proper nutrient and oxygen flow, Peter's respiratory, digestive, and nervous systems were compromised. These deficiencies can produce flaccid muscle tone or spastic muscles, depending on the individual, says Steiner. In Peter's case, the result was spasm. "His stomach and lungs, starved of the innervation, oxygen, and nutrients they needed, were having trouble expanding and contracting."

The Results of a Difficult Birth

Peter's birth had been a difficult one. It was a prolonged labor that after four days ended in the use of forceps. His head was twisted to one side as he came through the birth canal. After birth, he was removed to intensive care for the better part of a week and given antibiotics because he had an infection. The attendant congestion (called "wet lungs") prevented him from being able to breathe in a prone position unless his mother was nursing him.

Further examination revealed the structural source of Peter's restricted CSF flow. His traumatic birth had resulted in misalignment of his skull bones, with one overlapping the other, instead of being positioned side by side as is normal. The bones had remained in this compressed position rather than sliding back into place after passage through the birth canal. The result of the overlap was continual pressure inside Peter's head. His head-banging and face-hitting were likely attempts to relieve the pressure.

The temporal bones in his skull (the bones that the ears sit in) were compressed (medially) and lacked synchrony in their movement. Steiner gives a simplified explanation of the complex importance of the temporal bones in the craniosacral mechanism:

"The temporal bones are the active driving mechanism of the cranial system. The suture joints look like interdigitations or gears as they mesh and unmesh at the joints of the cranial vault. The temporals on their upper aspect have a beveled edge that slides and glides. The lower aspects of the temporal bones articulate with the sphenoid and the occiput. The suture joints at those contacts then propel the other bones.

"As the brain produces cerebrospinal fluid, the suture joints move away from each other in expansion to accomodate the increased fluid volume and pressure. This in turn causes a propulsion of the temporal bones. They open like gills of a fish, which allows for further production of CSF. When they get to the end range of motion, receptors in the suture joints signal to the brain, 'I can't go any further, I need to contract, it's too much.' The brain then lessens the production of cerebrospinal, allowing these bones to very slowly come back to what's called a 'closed-packed' position.

"At that point, the squeezing pressure of these bones on the sponge-like sinus around the brain circulates cerebrospinal fluid along the spinal cord and back up around the brain. This is the semi-closed hydraulic pumping mechanism. Then it all starts over again, where we're producing, producing, producing, everything's expanding, we get to that maximal expansion, and then we are retracting, retracting, retracting. Everything then is supporting the distribution of cerebrospinal fluid."

In Peter's case, his temporal bones were operating independently from each other, with one moving to accommodate the production phase, and the other the distribution phase. Steiner likens this situation to when the thermostat in your house malfunctions, and repeatedly clicks on, but the heat never rises. With the temporal bones not moving in synchrony, production and distribution of cerebrospinal fluid is reduced, which, as we have discussed, has repercussions throughout the body. As noted previously, a fixed coronal suture, which is the result of compressed temporal bones, is typical in many autisoid children.

Another source of Peter's compromised CSF flow was misalignment in his sacrum, which could also explain his walking problems and loss of coordination. Steiner explains that as time went on and the misalignments resulting from the traumatic birth went uncorrected, his body became less and less able to cope or compensate, and so his development regressed.

Intensive Therapy

Peter received CST (of which SER is a component) and Visceral Manipulation treatments, with three visits the first week and then two to four visits weekly over the next three months.

Through CST, the overlap in Peter's skull was corrected, and the accompanying pressure in his head released. "The results were immediate and dramatic," recalls Steiner. The head-banging and face-hitting ceased virtually immediately. To his mother's amazement, Peter lay still for his treatments for as long as two hours whereas before he had not been able to keep still for even ten minutes during medical procedures. After only two treatments, he slept through the night; that welcome development continued thereafter, with only a few exceptions.

Peter's other symptoms improved as well. After his first week of treatment, he started talking again and even using sentences. His eye contact increased, and he answered questions put to him, instead of responding with screams or odd noises. He also began eating more throughout the day; later, when Visceral Manipulation had helped improve his digestion, his food repertoire expanded.

After six weeks, Peter no longer looked wan and sickly. His face had filled out, and he had a rosier color. At the end of his treatment, his coordination was much better, he was walking again, and stimulation was less overwhelming to him. In addition, his chronic sinus congestion had disappeared.

In summarizing the changes in Peter, Steiner says: "I wasn't aware, when his parents first brought him in, of the depth of his dysfunction. It was only when his functions started to come back that I saw how much he had been a bright boy trapped in a body that wasn't working for him. I think his whole being was aware that he was somehow functioning at a lower decibel. He didn't take risks. He didn't venture out. Most kids aren't even aware of consequences. This little guy was aware that the world was unsafe for him on some level."

Certainly, his traumatic birth had sent that message to him.

Cellular Memory

The emotions of babies undergoing experiences like Peter's birth are often overlooked, as if someone so young doesn't feel the way an adult does in going through a traumatic event. Steiner states that it is clear by what occurs in patients when CranioSacral therapy becomes SomatoEmotional Release that infants are aware during birth and traumatized by experiences such as being delivered via the "battering ram" intensity of Pitocin (see chapter 8) or pulled out with forceps. When you consider what some infants go through to enter the world, it is difficult to come up with an equivalent occurrence in adult life—trapped and vulnerable, helpless, fighting for breath, survival threatened, yanked by the head or foot out of the birth canal.

Equally overlooked, both in babies and adults, is the storage in the body of the emotions felt during traumatic events. These emotional residues are the basis of what is known as cellular memory. The body remembers all the traumas—whether physical injury or emotional upset—an individual has experienced, because the attendant emotions are stored in its very tissues.

As explained in the earlier section on soma therapies, these emotional residues can be stored in energy cysts anywhere in the body. "The cellular memory in that energy cyst can be visual, kinesthetic, auditory, or 'all of the above,'" Steiner explains. As the emotions are released from the energy cysts during SER, patients reexperience the emotions and may even remember the event involved, such as the circumstances of their birth, along with sights, smells, and sounds accompanying that event.

As with all of the soma therapies, in SomatoEmotional Release the therapists take their cue from the patient's body. "We follow the body," explains Steiner, "If you were to feel in your own body the position that your body is inclined to go into, that would be the position that we would follow. Ultimately, the body would take us to the injury that caused the position, so at the depths of that movement pattern is the original injury. You might have a memory of it. You might say, 'Oh, this is the fall from the tricycle at age three.'"

In Peter's case, he nursed during a lot of the treatments. Nursing was the only thing that his mother had found would ease his sense of being overwhelmed, recalls Steiner. Although Peter's mother had provided the Centre with a complete written history, Steiner and the other hands-on therapists opted not to know the details of Peter's birth before seeing him. "We wanted the ability to be unbiased as we did our assessment of him," she explains. They only learned of the details of his birth as he assumed different positions on the table and his mother recognized what they were and explained to the therapists what was happening.

In this way, they learned the details of the traumatic event underlying Peter's physical and functional problems. In the process of spontaneously reenacting his birth, Peter released the emotional residues of the trauma, clearing the energy cysts in his body that were also contributing to his physical and functional imbalance.

After his treatment course, Peter's distortions and compressions had been corrected, his body had achieved a balance point, his organs were restored to healthy function, his energy cysts and their emotional content were cleared, and many of his autisoid manifestations had disappeared. Peter's mother entered him in a school for children with verbal delays. Two years later, he had caught up with his age group and showed no sign of ever having been autistic. To his mother's great joy and relief, he now ran and played happily like other children.

10 *The Tomatis Method: Listening and Autism*

Listening specialist Paul Madaule has been working with autistic children for 30 years, using the Tomatis Method to help them awaken to listening. In his view, a disorder in the ability to listen, which is distinct from hearing, is fundamental to the autistic condition.

Hearing, like seeing, is a passive act. Sounds, or sights, simply arrive at our ears, or eyes. Listening, like looking, however, requires action, intention, motivation, and focus, he explains. To listen to something, we have to focus our ears on the sound, just as in looking at something, we have to focus our eyes on the object. According to Madaule, a person with autism has an inner disconnection, a breakdown in communication, that interferes with his ability to focus in this way.

While autism as a communication problem is patently obvious to anyone acquainted with the disorder, Madaule is referring to something other than the outward manifestations of silence and withdrawal. "My point of view is that in the autistic child the communication problem is that he doesn't communicate with himself. He receives information from the outside as in sight, sound, and touch, but he doesn't have a sense of himself."

Without a sense of self, the child has no way to organize or understand the sights, sounds, and tactile sensations he is receiving, thus the confusing and often overwhelming bombardment of the senses that autistic individuals have reported. Aptly, Madaule uses a music metaphor to illustrate the problem. "If the different senses were musical instruments, in autism those instruments lack a conductor. They are not able to play something together, which permits you to move toward higher function, particularly language function. In the Tomatis view, the ear is the conductor. When I speak of the ear, I mean the sensory organ *and* all its connections to the nervous system and the whole body."[189]

What Is the Tomatis Method?

A sensory integration technique, the Tomatis Method is listening training via sound stimulation. It is a remedial intervention for auditory processing disorders, attentional problems, learning disabilities, language delays, and communication problems, such as those found in autistic spectrum disorders. Developed by French physician Alfred A. Tomatis in the early 1950s, it arose from his work in helping opera singers improve their voice control and range.

The sound and music filtering device he invented, called the Electronic Ear, became the centerpiece of his method and is highly useful as an ear training tool for children with developmental delays and disorders, such as autism and learning disabilities. Dr. Tomatis defines the Electronic Ear as a "simulator of high quality listening."[190]

Helping the child learn to listen is a means of effecting sensory integration and of awakening the child to a sense of self, of bringing him back home, if you will. This enables him to integrate his inner world, which then translates into an ability to communicate and connect with the outer world.

More specifically, it is a sound-amplification and sound-filtering system that randomly modifies the frequency content of the sound source, which can be music or voice. Sound is received in a pulsative mode, the pur-

Potential Benefits of the Tomatis Method

The following improvements may occur with the use of the Tomatis Method in cases of autism:[191]

- improved language skills
- use of "I" to refer to the self, instead of using the third person
- increased desire to communicate
- improved social skills
- initiation of social contact
- follows directions better
- less aggressive behavior
- less repetitive behavior
- better eye contact
- more interest in people and surroundings
- improved listening skills
- better sensory integration
- decreased hypersensitivity to sound
- fewer temper tantrums
- longer attention span
- reduced tactile defensiveness
- increased affect
- more affectionate
- improved appreciation for food
- less picky eating
- can be toilet trained
- better self-image

pose of which is to exercise the ear. Listening training thus gives the ear a good "earobic" workout.[192] The person undergoing the training wears headphones attached by a long cord to the Electronic Ear. In the case of children, this means they can move about freely and play while receiving the training.

The Tomatis Method is based on the premise that improving listening by exercising the ear and stimulating the nervous system with recorded and filtered sound improves learning, language, and communication skills, as well as social interaction abilities.

Helping the child learn to listen is a means of effecting sensory integration and of awakening the child to a sense of self, of bringing him back home, if you will. This enables him to integrate his inner world, which then translates into an ability to communicate and connect with the outer world. Madaule, director of the Listening Centre in Toronto, Canada, which is the oldest Tomatis center in North America, has seen listening training bring about these changes in many children. Thirty to forty autistic children come to the Centre every year.

Currently, there are twenty-one Tomatis centers in North America, and some 200 around the world.

While the word "training" may summon images of instruction and the arduous task of forcing a child to pay attention, the reality of the Tomatis Method is quite different. If you walk into a child's listening session, what you will see is a playroom in which a child wearing headphones is drawing, painting, playing with toys, or interacting with other children or the listening therapist. The sound coming through the headphones is usually Mozart or a recording of the mother's voice. Music and voice are filtered or pure, based on assessment of the child, and changed as the child moves through the developmental stages of listening. As the ear and brain are the direct recipients of the sound stimulation, the child does not need to focus on the sound and can engage in other activities while the training transpires.

The story of Timmy reveals what listening training can do for autism.

Timmy: *Coming Out of* His *Shell*

Timmy started the program at the Listening Centre when he was three and a half years old, just after receiving a diagnosis of PDD (pervasive developmental disorder). He had been a quiet baby, according to his mother. In fact, she described him as a "dream child," especially in contrast to his demanding younger brother, who was born not long after Timmy. She didn't see anything wrong in the beginning, but delayed motor functions and speech raised the alarm.

At three and a half, Timmy was locked inside himself, oblivious to his surroundings. His mother reported that he still had not spoken, had trouble understanding, found it difficult to participate in most activities, showed no interest in his peers, displayed no socialization, and was not toilet trained. He also constantly had bruises from bumping into things. He did show feelings in crying or laughing, however, and was affectionate, which indi-

> **In Their Own Words**
>
> *"Our little guy was like a walking zombie. He had no facial expressions. He had no interest in anybody. He couldn't differentiate between a live person and an object... He was just in his own little realm. He never hugged us. No communications. Nothing. Everyone we went to told us the same thing: He would probably be that way for the rest of his life."*
>
> *After only the early stages of listening training, Eric is beginning to verbalize. "He plays with toys now. He never played with toys before. His neurologist just couldn't believe the changes in him. This neurologist...[had] basically told us there was nothing for Eric."*[193]
>
> —mother of Eric, 3

cated that he was not totally disconnected. Timmy was what Madaule calls the "hypo type" of autistic, the more traditional autism. He was very quiet and it was easy to take him places, unlike a child of the "hyper type," which is characterized by behavior problems and prolonged tantrums.

After the first week in his initial 30 hours of listening training (two hours daily for 15 days), Timmy was more receptive, his balance was better, and he had stopped bumping into things, which indicated improvement in his sensory motor function. After the second week, he was more mischievous, getting into trouble, and demanding more attention, all of which Madaule regards as a positive sign. "You could see the child had really come out of his shell," he says. "We are trying to develop his ego, his sense of himself. His sense of self starts with the ability to say 'no,' which is very much what happens with a young child at two to three years old. I say 'no,' therefore I exist."

Madaule is careful to prepare parents beforehand for these changes in behavior and explain to them why it is good news when their autistic child starts getting into trouble. It is also important to communicate this information to any other people working with the child, such as those doing ABA (Applied Behavior Analysis) or other behavior management interventions.

If they aren't forewarned of the potential changes, they may conclude the child is getting worse, unwittingly quash the child's new-found ego, and discourage the parents from continuing with listening training.

While many people come to the Listening Centre from far away, Timmy lived in Toronto, so continued with his usual life during the training. After the second week, his mother reported that Timmy had started to draw faces, said a few words, and wanted to help and participate at home. His bruises were disappearing, with no new ones added. His school reported that he was more "there," seemed more with it, and was responding more to other children. He wasn't running round and round, in complete nonrelation to the other children, the way he used to. He showed improvement in art, too, drawing more easily. This, along with the fact that he was no longer bumping into things, indicated better coordination, which in turn reflects a clearer body image and a stronger sense of self.

After the first 30 hours of the program, Timmy had a month off before the second round to give his mind and body time to integrate the changes put into motion by the listening training. Madaule notes that more profound changes often occur in between listening sessions than during them, as the child incorporates the input. In a progress review before starting the second set of 30 hours, Timmy's parents reported that all the previous gains had been maintained. He was also now responding to directions and more aware of the *do*s and *don't*s. He didn't obey systematically, however, a reflection of the "I say 'no,' therefore I am" pattern. He was more interested in other kids and shared more. Acknowledgment of the self and acknowledgment of others work together, says Madaule. If you don't acknowledge yourself, you are not going to be able to acknowledge others.

Timmy was also more spontaneous, which is difficult for children who become upset at departure from routine and ritual, as is the case with many autistic children. Timmy's teacher observed that he was initiating play with other children, and his speech therapist reported that he had a longer attention span. He showed greater interest in letters and numbers and had begun to chatter, with a few real words amidst the nonsense words. Jargonism, the chatter of nonsense words, is an important stage in the development of language, notes Madaule. It is the step after babble and precedes actual sentences.

At the end of the next 30 hours of listening training, Timmy was spelling his name, being more assertive, expressing emotion more, and attempting to communicate, not just engaging in jargonism or echolalia (parroting others).

Thereafter, Timmy came back to the Centre every six months for a 10-hour booster. In the review before starting the first booster (nine months after he had started the program), Timmy's parents reported that he had begun talking—much more at school than at home. Home is a place where the children know they can be understood without having to speak, so it is quite usual for them to talk more at school, says Madaule.

Although Timmy's speech was not yet age-appropriate, he was initiating conversation, which is an important development, in that it signals the understanding of and the desire to communicate and also is a departure from autistic passivity. He was initiating expressions of affection more, too, holding a hand or giving a kiss. This emotional interaction is also important, says Madale, as autistics may interact, but it is often without emotional content.

According to his mother, Timmy seemed to be making "a conscious effort to come out of his shell." His behavior outside of the house was appropriate, and he was playing with toys more appropriately, meaning recognizing a toy for the object it represented and using it as such, as in moving a toy truck as though it is driving. "Being able to play with the toy is to be able to start using your imagination, which is what these children are not able to do," says Madaule. "They are very much into the factual, the concrete."

Timmy was also making progress in toilet training. In Madaule's view, the delay in this area relates to delayed speech. "Toilet training is very much connected to language acquisition," he says. "It is common for kids who have delayed language—speaking problems, learning disabilities, difficulty reading and writing—to have toilet control issues." According to Dr. Tomatis, the same nerve (the vagus nerve) that innervates the larynx has neural connections with the bladder and rectum. This nerve also has a sensory branch in the eardrum. By stimulating the ear, listening training improves larynx control and may also influence sphincter function relating to toilet habits because of its action on the vagus nerve.

With only biannual boosters, Timmy's progress continued over the next five years. At the age of nine and a half, he was in the fourth grade, engaging in conversation, and doing very well. He got a B-plus in math and wrote a three-page book report, which he read to his class. Although he was far more adaptable, he still showed some of the rigidity and inflexibility of compulsive tendencies, wanting everything to be perfect and getting upset when it wasn't, as well as overfocusing on people's watches and clothes.

Now 10 years old, Timmy is in a normal grade level, although it is a struggle. His biggest problem is still social adjustment, reports Madaule. "The role of therapists, educators, and parents is to make sure he has all the communication tools he needs when he is ready to open up and be part of the social realm, which often happens at puberty."

Timmy's motor function is good now, he prints and types well, but writing cursive is difficult for him. His fine motor skill is still not there and might never be, says Madaule, "but thank God we have technology that permits us to overcome that." (Timmy is quite comfortable with the computer.) Timmy's speech still needs work. Lacking intonation and flow, it sounds somewhat robotic at this point. The speech therapist and further listening training can refine his speech, notes Madaule, so the robotic aspect could change with time.

On Timmy's last visit to the Centre, he told a story extemporaneously that his mother wrote down for him. "On Sunday, I'm going to Turks and Caicos Islands. I will go on an airplane. Airplanes are noisy. The engines are loud. I can wear my earplugs. I can listen to music with headphones. It is very loud when we take off from the ground and later when we land." Then he drew a picture to accompany the story.

This was a very different child from the one who had walked into the Centre six and a half years before. "He went from a moderate-to-severe form of autism to a mild form," says Madaule. The changes in Timmy occurred with only 90 hours of listening training (9 boosters of 10 hours each at 6-month intervals) after the initial 60 hours.

For information about Tomatis centers around the world, see the Tomatis website (www.tomatis.com).

How the Tomatis Method Works

Over three decades ago, Paul Madaule sought the help of Dr. Tomatis for his problems with dyslexia, which today would be diagnosed as ADD with learning disabilities, he comments. He was so impressed with the technique and its results that he devoted himself to working with Dr. Tomatis, and in 1978 opened the Listening Centre.

Although the Tomatis Method is used for many conditions as well as simply improving singing and listening skills, it is particularly known for its benefits for autism and learning disabilities. The population for which it is most helpful could be summarized simply as those with listening problems. Listening problems fall on a continuum, explains Madaule. The continuum ranges from language-related learning disabilities on one end—"These are partial, mild listening problems, which translate into problems learning to read, learning to write, and learning to express, oral language problems," he says—to the more severe end, with severe language and communication problems, autistic-like problems.

From a listening standpoint, a person with a learning disability has a distortion in his listening ability and an autistic person is disconnected from what he listens to, says Madaule. "Both may hear fine. But those with autism are not only *not* processing, as is the case with the learning disabled, they are not connecting what they hear with themselves." This is the point made earlier about a breakdown in communication with the self.

In considering this breakdown more closely, you can discover much in the behavior of autistic children that signals inner disconnection. One example is the characteristic practice of autistic children to refer to themselves in the third person (he/she or by their name), or sometimes the second person (you); they don't typically say "I." It is as though they are perceiving themselves from the outside, notes Madaule. The disconnection reveals itself in the way they relate to the world around them, too. Not recognizing themselves as a person, they don't recognize others as people. "They don't seem to distinguish the difference between a person or an object, a puppet or a pet."

To explain what all this has to do with listening, it's necessary to review the function of the ear. The inner ear consists of two sensory receptors: the vestibule, or vestibular system, and the cochlea. The vestibule (a double cavity with three appending tubes, resembling a bagpipe) is responsible for balance and the perception of gravity and the body's position and movement in space; it also plays a role in maintaining muscle tone. The vestibule is connected to the cochlea, a spiral shell-like structure responsible for sound reception. The vestibule is also connected via nerve pathways to the cerebellum, the area of the brain involved in regulation of motor function.

Madaule suggests that the self-stimulating behaviors characteristic of autistic children—spinning, rocking, hand flapping in front of the face—are "indications of an attempt to stimulate the vestibular system, which is not working."

An indication that children with autism have a problem in their vestibular system is the fact that they often lack what is called postrotatory nystagmus, which is the normal eye movement response to the body being rotated. Nystagmus is the involuntary movement of the eyeball, and evidences the influence of the vestibular system on eye movement. A good example of postrotatory nystagmus occurs after a child spins round and round, as children love to do to make themselves dizzy so they can watch the world spin round them when they stop.

Normally, after this activity, the eyes move back and forth and the child weaves when she tries to walk. In the autistic child, there is no eye movement and she can walk a straight line after spinning. Madaule suggests that the self-stimulating behaviors characteristic of autistic children—spinning, rocking, hand flapping in front of the face—are "indications of an attempt to stimulate the vestibular system, which is not working."

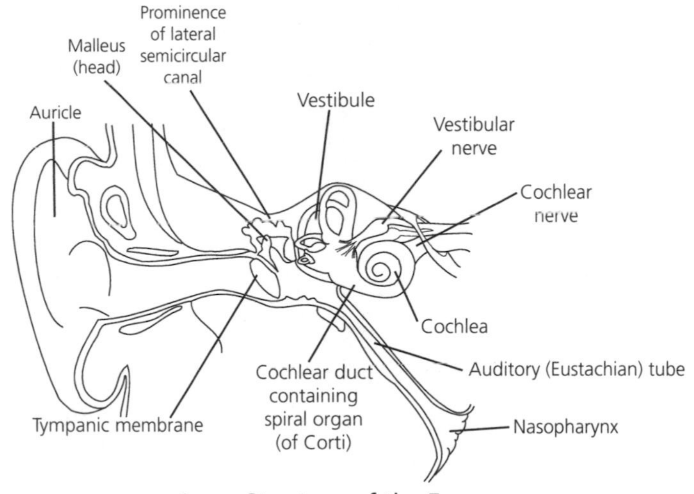

Inner Structure of the Ear

The links begin to become clear with the following fact: "This vestibular system is part of what makes us aware of our body in space, that helps us to identify ourselves as an 'I,'" says Madaule. "This is why I like to call the vestibular system the 'ear of the body.'" The Tomatis Method seeks to reestablish the connection to self, the sense of "I," by stimulating both the auditory (cochlea) and the vestibular systems with sound.

One of the great contributions of Dr. Tomatis was to describe the relationship between the cochlear system, the mechanism of hearing, and the vestibular system, the mechanism of balance and

The Infant Ear

The hearing of a newborn is fully operational at birth. In fact, from between five and six months in the womb, the baby is hearing. The acoustic nerve is the first nerve in the body to be myelinized, which means that it can then transmit nerve impulses, or messages. The myelin sheath is the covering on nerves that enables these messages to travel along the nerve.

Not only is the child in utero hearing, but she is also listening. She "reaches" out her ear to catch the sound of her mother's voice over the other noises that come through to her in the womb, says Paul Madaule. "That is the first attempt at listening." The goal of the sound stimulation program at the Listening Centre is to awaken that early desire to listen, "to make the children want to reach out from behind their sensory shells, to ignite their desire to hear."[194]

movement perception, which conventional medicine tends to regard as two separate, distinct systems. "In fact, this connection is well known to anyone who dances. Dancing to different kinds of music naturally induces different kinds of body movements," says Madaule.

On a physiological level, if you consider the fluids of the ear, the connection is also evident. The endolymphatic fluid that is inside the cochlea is also inside the vestibular system, he notes. "The fluid is stimulated by sound, when the ear receives sound, and also by movement, when we move, which gives us a sense of movement. Now, what's interesting, just a point of anatomy, is that the same fluid is shared by the two systems. This is not two systems. It's one system." This explains why the sound stimulation of listening training has such far-reaching effects, improving not only listening-related skills, but also coordination, balance, and ultimately the sense of self and others.

The implications of vestibular problems are sweeping. For language development, both oral and written, the child needs both the sound and the body components, says Madaule. To produce sounds, one has to use the body. Autistic children's disconnection from their bodies is one of the reasons why they don't speak, he notes. Further, Tomatis pointed out that the same nerves (the vagus and others) are involved in both voice production and control of the middle ear muscles, evidence of the close link between listening and speaking.[195]

Repatterning Listening

The purpose of listening training is to repattern the listening ability. This is accomplished by taking children through all the developmental stages of listening, from the very beginning, with the aim that this reliving and reprogramming of the stages will allow them to make up for anything they might have missed. Taking the child back to the first listening in the womb (see sidebar, "The Infant Ear") begins the process.

For this, the child hears the filtered voice of the mother. Filtering out the lower frequencies in the recorded voice of the mother reproduces the way sounds are heard in the womb, according to Dr. Tomatis.[196] "What we are trying to do with his mother's voice is to give what I call the music of language, the basic rhythm and melody of the language to which the child later adds the words," says Madaule, likening the mother's voice to a blueprint of language in the child's brain.

The child also listens to Mozart, unfiltered at first, which means the entire music spectrum is present. Mozart is the music of choice because Dr. Tomatis discovered that it was the most universally appealing. The appeal truly is universal: "In all traditional or pre-modern societies where different Western music is introduced, the music of Mozart is the only one that is always accepted," states Madaule.[197] It is also the only music Dr. Tomatis found "that creates a perfect balance between the charging effect and a sense of calmness and well-being."[198] It relaxes or energizes as needed.

The other music the Tomatis Method employs is Gregorian chant. It is used when the child is overly anxious, hyperactive, or hypersensitive. The chant exerts a calming influence. Listening training also uses children's songs and dances to promote vestibular system activity.

For later developmental stages of listening, the lower frequencies are filtered out by the Electronic Ear device. The filtering of the music is to train the ear to discriminate sounds precisely at all the levels of the auditory spectrum. The program emphasizes full-spectrum music for quite a long time with autistic children because the low frequencies have the most impact on the vestibular system, explains Madaule. The full spectrum stimulates the whole ear, but specifically the vestibule. "Low frequencies are those that make us become more aware of our body and of the movement of the body. They ground us."

When the child has achieved this grounding, the lower frequencies are filtered out and the medium frequencies emphasized. The middle range, which is the range specific to language sounds, facilitates the development of language. Gradually, the filtering progresses to leave only the high frequencies, which relate to mental ability, attention, and concentration, according to Madaule. The high range is energizing as well, while the lower range promotes relaxation. "One of the principles of the work of Tomatis is never to cut the high frequency because, for all this to be integrated, we need to constantly stimulate the nervous system. That is what the high frequency helps you to do. Even if you want to work on the body (low range), you also want the brain to be able to integrate what you're doing,"

Consistent with this developmental approach, after working on receptive listening (listening to recorded music and the mother's voice), the method works on audio-vocal control. This entails the child using a microphone, which permits him to hear his own voice when babbling, singing, and talking. "The purpose is to complete and reinforce the ear-voice control loop, which is key in language development," Madaule explains.

Typically, listening training begins and ends with the full spectrum, with all the filtered levels delivered in between. The ideal schedule is a first series of sound stimulation for two hours a day for 15 days (a total of 30 hours), followed by a month's break, then another 15 days (30 hours), and after that boosters of 10 hours over 5 days every 3 (or sometimes every 6) months.

A Listening Checklist

The listening skills or level of a person cannot be assessed directly, but must be determined through related skills and behavior, as well as a consideration of developmental history, which may reveal conditions or events that cause listening problems. If a number of the items below apply to an individual, that person may have a listening problem.

Developmental History

This knowledge is extremely important in early identification and prevention of listening problems. It also sheds light on the possible causes.

- a stressful pregnancy
- difficult birth
- early separation from the mother
- adoption
- delay in motor development
- recurring ear infections

Receptive Listening

This is the listening that is directed outward. It keeps us attuned to the world around us, to what's going on at home, at work, or in the classroom.

- short attention span
- distractibility
- oversensitivity to sounds
- misinterpretation of questions
- confusion of similar sounding words
- frequent need of repetition
- inability to follow sequential instructions

Motor Skills

The ear of the body, which controls balance, coordination, and body image, also needs close attention.

- poor posture
- fidgety behavior
- clumsy, uncoordinated movement
- poor sense of rhythm
- messy handwriting
- hard time with organization, structure
- confusion of left and right
- mixed dominance
- poor sport skills

A Listening Checklist (continued)

Energy Level

The ear acts as a dynamo, providing us with the energy we need to survive and lead fulfilling lives.

- difficulty getting up
- tiredness at the end of the day
- habit of procrastinating
- hyperactivity
- tendency toward depression
- feeling overburdened with everyday tasks

Expressive Listening

This is listening that is directed within. We use it to control our voice when we speak and sing.

- flat and monotonous voice
- hesitant speech
- weak vocabulary
- poor sentence structure
- overuse of stereotyped expressions
- inability to sing in tune
- confusion or reversal of letters
- poor reading comprehension
- poor reading aloud
- poor spelling

Behavioral and Social Adjustment

A listening difficulty is often related to these:

- low tolerance of frustration
- poor self-confidence
- poor self-image
- shyness
- difficulty making friends
- tendency to withdraw, avoid others
- irritability
- immaturity
- low motivation, no interest in school/work
- negative attitude toward school/work

Source: Reprinted with permission of Paul Madaule and The Listening Centre, Toronto, Ontario, Canada, © 1998.

The interim between the sound stimulation sets is a continuation of the therapy, "a time for incubation, a time for rumination." Madaule likens it to what happens during sleep. "During the night, you solve the problems of the day. This is the same thing, except that it takes a little bit more time to integrate 15 days of 30 hours of stimulation." For people who travel long distances to the Centre, it can be a hardship to take the breaks between the sessions, but the integration can't be rushed. "We are trying to reproduce a step in development, and development takes time and requires periods of rest. You can't do this all at once because that's not the way development works."

Sean: Becoming the Child He Was Meant to Be

Sean came to the Listening Centre from a country in northern Africa. He was seven years old and had a severe form of autism. Prior to his diagnosis at three years old, doctors had run auditory tests because he behaved as though he was deaf. Sean had never spoken. (Madaule notes that most of the autistic children he sees had begun to talk and then regressed.) In Sean's case, it was difficult for his parents to understand what he wanted. He didn't have the ability to tell them, even with gestures such as pointing or other nonverbal means.

While he would not engage in eye contact and was socially withdrawn, he was more of the hyper type of autism, screaming at the top of his lungs and showing hypersensitivity to sound and touch. Like most autistic children, he was extremely rigid in how things needed to be done. He would throw terrible temper tantrums when things didn't go his way. His tactile defensiveness manifested in not wanting to be touched, have his hair cut, or his have teeth brushed. He also showed digestive sensitivity, ate little, and was an extremely picky eater when he did eat. He didn't sleep well either.

Sean's story is an especially good illustration of what listening training can accomplish because he comes from a country where very little is done for autistic children, according to Madaule. After the initial 30 hours of sound stimulation, the family returned home and continued with exactly what they had been doing before, which was nothing more than a little bit of occupational and speech therapy. The services available to them were limited, and they didn't implement a special diet or the other interventions people in North America typically try. As a result, the effects of listening training were more clearcut than in other cases.

Although Sean was unaware of the world around him, he could walk with ease on a wall seven feet high, only eight inches wide, his parents reported. Perhaps he could do this with no difficulty *because* he was unaware and had no fear or concept of consequences. In any case, he obviously didn't have the balance and motor coordination problems that Timmy had. This illustrates that the vestibular system in autistic children can work well in one area, such as balance, but not in those areas related to communication, as indicated by lack of eye contact and no pointing.

Sean had the usual 2 hours a day of sound stimulation for 15 days. For the first 10 hours, he listened to nonfiltered Mozart, and then a sound stimulation "cocktail" of progressingly filtered music in half-hour periods alternating with half-hour periods of his mother's voice, also filtered.

After the first week (15 hours), he was engaging in some eye contact, an amazing and welcome eventuality for his parents. Sean demonstrated some control of his impulses, meaning that when he was told not to do something, instead of throwing a tantrum right away, he would wait for a few seconds.

After the second week (30 hours), there was more modulation in his voice and "richer jargonism," which meant that he was attempting to produce vocalizations that sounded like language. As noted previously, jargonism is an important developmental step in language. "Even if he's seven years old, he has to go through this step," states Madaule. Sean was also obeying more easily and quickly. This indicated mental adaptability and that he was paying attention, both of which require receptive listening skills.

A month later, in the review before the second session, Sean's parents reported that he had started to repeat the first syllables of words. After seven years of not speaking, he was beginning to develop some language after only 30 hours of sound stimulation.

He was also more observant of the world around him, showing curiosity, and had become interested in playing the piano, a sign of the wakening of auditory discrimination, says Madaule.

At the same time, he had become more autonomous; for example, he would take off his clothes and wash himself on his own, instead of passively sitting and waiting for his mother to come and do it. He had started smiling and responded to humor on television, neither of which is characteristic of people with autism. "Autistic children tend to think literally and consequently do not have a sense of humor," Madaule observes.

During the 30 hours of the second visit, Sean was obviously more aware of his surroundings, looking around and observing what was happening. He also showed respect for other people's space, which meant that he had a better sense of his own space, comments Madaule. He exhibited more awareness of the consequences of his actions. His ability and willingness to maintain eye contact continued to improve. He could now say a few basic, but real, words in the appropriate context, such as good-bye when leaving and good night when going to bed. Again, this was after seven years of no words.

In Their Own Words

"Every time [Jordan] would get angry he would just smash his head on the floor. . . . He would hurt the other kids. He'd bite and scratch. . . . The doctors told us he would never get better. He might have to be institutionalized. He might never talk. There was no light at the end of the tunnel. It was just doom, doom, doom. I kept thinking, 'What am I going to do when he is sixteen and bigger than I am?'"

After a year of listening training, life is almost normal for Jordan and his family. Now three and a half, he can speak, read, and write. "Doctors still tell us he's autistic and there's no cure. Paul says in two years the word autism will be a faded memory [for us]. I tend to believe Paul because everything he's said has come true."[199]

—mother of Jordan

Sean's parents noted that all of his sensitivities—tactile, auditory, and gustatory—disappeared quickly, within two to three months after he began listening training.

Following the second thirty-hour set of sound stimulation, Madaule recommended a home program. For this, the child uses a LiFT (Listening Fitness Trainer) machine, designed at the Listening Centre. About the size of a Walkman, it is a miniature battery-run audio device, programmed with sound/music tailored to the individual. With this technology, it is now possible to continue the listening training at home.

For information about LiFT, see the websites www.listeningfitness.com or www.listeningcentre.com, or contact the Listening Centre in Toronto, Canada: 416-588-4136 or listen@idirect.com.

When Sean came back to the Centre for the third time, it was 10 months after his last visit and he had done 20 hours of the home program in the interval. He was eight years old by then and looked and behaved very much like a boy of his age. Madaule explains what this means: "Children who are severely autistic tend to become more and more age inappropriate as time goes on. A behavior that might be funny or cute at four years old is not funny or cute at seven years old." Sean was changing as his autism shifted from severe to mild.

"He was more aware, more in the here and now," reports Madaule. He was able to repeat about 20 words, but beyond words he had more means to express himself and was able to make his needs understood. He now had some interests—in fact a wide range—and had let his parents know that he wanted to do karate, play tennis, go to a swimming pool, and have a scooter. With the gustative sensitivity gone, he ate everything. His stereotypic movements, such as hand fluttering, had disappeared, except in cases of extreme excitement. He asked for kisses and could now be playful. Able to engage in imaginative play, he would use a toy as the object it represented.

The parents were very excited to report that, for the first

time, they could go on a vacation with Sean to a hotel because his behavior now permitted it. The tantrums, throwing food, and refusing to sit had all disappeared. In a public place, he also now watched for where his parents were. Before, they had to hold his hand constantly—to which he objected strenuously—to keep him from running off and getting lost. In addition, Sean had developed patience and was able to sit and wait, in the waiting room at the Centre, for example. "Last year, you could not have even thought of that," says Madaule. "Just realizing the parents were not around, he would have thrown a temper tantrum."

Sean also demonstrated a willingness to participate in family activity, something which previously did not interest him. Before, he would not do anything that didn't give him gratification, which is typical of not having social skills. Further, he would make an effort to do something instead of being passive. For example, instead of sitting and waiting for someone to lace his shoes, he would try to do it himself. "His attempt may be reduced by the difficulty and perhaps attention span, which is still a little bit short, but at least there is an attempt," observes Madaule. "There is no learning possible if there is no attempt."

Madaule recommended that the parents put Sean in a mainstream school, so he would have appropriate behavior models. "These kids learn a lot by imitation," he says. "What can a child learn if he spends his day with children who are functioning at a lower level than he is? There are no models there." One of the goals of listening training is to bring the children to the point where they can be integrated. "Integration with peers in a regular setting is one of the best things that can happen to an autistic child. But the child has to be open enough to benefit from this social interaction." Listening training had brought Sean to that stage of opening.

Sean had 30 hours of sound stimulation on his third visit. Since he was severely autistic and an older child when he commenced the listening training, he needed more hours than the standard initial sixty followed by boosters. During the training, Madaule observed that Sean's words were more intelligible and that he had become quite good at explaining things by mimicking, much in the manner of a deaf-mute child. He was very specific about the toys he wanted to play with, indicating development of a connection with self.

Madaule is uncertain how far Sean is going to be able to progress in the development of language. "The blueprint of speech is very difficult to establish in the brain at eight years old, but we keep trying." Even with very limited speech, Sean has made tremendous gain. "Through the program, he acquired communications skills, which in the realm of things is more important than speech," says Madaule. He notes that deaf-mutes have no problem relating and communicating, aside from the limitations of not having speech or hearing. Sean is now in a similar situation. He no longer has the communication problem of disconnection from himself; he just doesn't use language as a means of communication yet.

Prelanguage, the understanding of communication, is perhaps the main benefit of the Tomatis Method for autistic children. With this understanding, they realize what something as simple as pointing means, a mental connection that eluded them before. The world of communication opens up to them.

Sean will continue his training via the LiFT machine, and Madaule hopes to see him until the beginning of adolescence. To summarize where Sean has arrived at this point, Madaule repeats what Sean's parents said: "He is really with us now. We really have the feeling that we have a child who is our son, who is the brother of our daughter."

The Importance of Prelanguage

When Madaule says that Sean developed communication skills through listening training, he is referring to the world of prelanguage. As discussed earlier in the chapter, the problem is not just that the autistic child doesn't talk, but, more seriously, that the child doesn't communicate, doesn't connect. This signals that the child lacks prelanguage skills, which are the nonverbal means of communication. Eye contact is one of the most significant of these; facial expression that indicates "I understand what you are saying" is another. The autistic child typically does not engage in eye contact or other attempts at communication. "Not only is he nonverbal, he's also non-nonverbal," observes Madaule.

As noted previously, the autistic child is disconnected from self, and therefore others. Communication is all about connecting. Without a sense of connection, there is no understanding of, or motivation for, communication. "Language needs a communication component. What is language about if I don't know what communication is about? The child is not connecting to the meaning. It's just words."

Prelanguage, the understanding of communication, is perhaps the main benefit of the Tomatis Method for autistic children. With this understanding, they realize what something as simple as pointing means, a mental connection that eluded them before. They can point at what they want and use other nonverbal expressions and gestures to make themselves understood. The world of communication opens up to them.

The first step in establishing prelanguage is eye contact, states Madaule. "It says, 'I'm with you. I'm in the here and now.' Eye contact is listening with the eyes." Listening training fosters eye contact through stimulating the vestibular system and regrounding the child, bringing him into his body, making him more "together," more present to himself. If he is more present to himself, he is more present to others. From there, he proceeds to a greater interest in others and starts playing with other children, a sibling first perhaps. "Playing is a communication skill," says Madaule. "When you see children who start to play, you already are a big step ahead." Looking at themselves in a mirror, something most autistic children don't do, is another indication of progress in prelanguage development, a sign that connection is happening.

The success of the program needs to be considered in relationship to the precise goals set for an individual child at the outset, states Madaule. The goals vary from child to child according to his

Auditory Integration Training (AIT)

Another form of sensory integration employing sound is Auditory Integration Training (AIT), well known for its application to autism. Developed by French doctor Guy Berard after he worked with Dr. Tomatis in the late 1950s, AIT has been used beneficially with conditions involving sensory input disturbances, including, in addition to classic autism: PDD, ADD, dyslexia, learning disabilities, Tourette's disorder, and Rett's disorder, among others.

According to Dr. Berard, AIT works by exercising the muscles in the middle ear. This stimulates areas of the brain relating to auditory pathways, which aids in normalizing the brain's response to sensory input and thus improves the body's reaction to sensory overload. As with the Tomatis Method, benefits from AIT may include improved language, more social interaction, more appropriate social behaviors, calmness, improved motor coordination, better balance, longer attention span, and less distractibility.

The core of the AIT program is 10 hours of listening to specially prepared music in half-hour sessions administered twice daily for 10 days. The program may be repeated multiple times. Like the Tomatis Method, the music has had specific frequencies filtered out, according to the particular needs of the individual, but the filtering technology and focus is different. The sound is delivered via devices known as the Audiokinetron or the Digital Auditory Aerobics machine.[200]

For more information on Auditory Integration Training, see the website www.aitresources.com.

age and the nature and severity of his problem. "There is a golden rule in working with children with language and communication problems: the earlier the better," he says. He urges parents to consult a listening training practitioner when their child is two years old if they perceive problems, instead of waiting for a formal diagnosis, which typically doesn't happen until the child is at least three. "This is usually a year and a half or longer after the onset of symptoms," notes Madaule, adding that the sooner treatment is started, the more effective it will be.

In general, with children who start at two to three years old, listening training can achieve very good and sometimes spectacular results, Madaule says. With children from four to six years old, results are often very good; with children older than that, the results tend not to be as good, but that is not always the case. Consider Sean, who began listening training at age seven.

In terms of the success rate regarding prelanguage skills, 80 to 90 percent of the children develop them. These skills include nonverbal communication skills, communication intent, the desire to communicate, flexibility, spontaneity, socialization, playfulness, expression of affect, and a longer attention span. Some children evidence vocalization or production of words, but that does not necessarily evolve into language.

Another golden rule with autism, says Madaule, is that listening training gets better results if the child talked and then lost speech than if the child never spoke. As a general measure of success for all the children, listening training—especially because it enhances prelanguage skills—prepares them for more traditional forms of intervention, both therapeutic and educational. "Our work greatly facilitates the work of more conventional interventions, speech therapy in particular. The child is ready now because he understands what language is all about," he says.

Observations on Autism and Listening

Paul Madaule's experience with autism echoes what many other health-care practitioners are saying. He, too, has seen autism increasing "very significantly" in the past 10 years, but it is a certain kind that is on the rise. "I have not seen an increase in the severely autistic, the ones we always called autistic. What is increasing is what we were calling before the autistic tendency. We now call it the autistic spectrum disorder, or PDD," he says.

He notes that a high proportion of these children seem to develop more or less well—perhaps not great, but all right—until about 18 months, and then they "go down." Madaule has recently begun gathering data on the immunization history of his autism patients. He suspects that when he compiles the data, he will see a correlation with vaccines and the onset of autistic symptoms, which could explain why the children tend to regress at around the same age.

In terms of the therapies that are often applied to autism, Madaule cautions against exclusive use of ABA (Applied Behavior Analysis). In his experience, it works best in combination with sensory integration, which he regards as a must for autistic children. There are two types of nonmedical interventions, he explains. The first type is the interventions that "are trying to get the child to 'receive,' to understand, to experience something within in order to express it out." Sensory integration methods such as listening training fall in this category.

The second type is behavioristic, rote training, such as ABA, that uses positive reinforcement to elicit speech and condition the child to behave in certain ways. "The child is going to say hello, good-bye, a few words, but he is going to say them because he's been conditioned to," comments Madaule. He notes that results are achieved with this type of technique, as statistics show, but it requires working with the child 30 to 40 hours a week. His objection to using this method alone is: "Does the child really get involved, humanistically speaking—or another way to say it, from the inside out—in what he's doing, or does he just react to what he's asked to do?"

By combining the two types of nonmedical intervention, you can do the behavioral management while helping to give the child a sense of himself. "Then he knows better what he's doing," says Madaule. Rather than ABA, however, he prefers to recommend an intervention called "floor time," developed by Stanley I. Greenspan, M.D. "I would like to see this more friendly and child-oriented approach, which fosters spontaneity, affect, prelanguage, and sensory integration, become more widely accepted."

For information about Floor Time, see Infancy and Early Childhood: The Practice of Clinical Assessment and Intervention with Emotional and Developmental Challenges, by Stanley I. Greenspan, M.D. (Madison, CT: International Universities Press, 1992); or visit his website at www.stanleygreenspan.com.

The practitioners delivering the different types of interventions need to keep each other informed, as illustrated by the earlier example of how deleterious it can be for the child—and family—if the behavior management practitioner is not told that behavior may worsen at first with listening training. Another example is that the gains children have made with listening training sometimes start to slip—eye contact may become less frequent, they may become withdrawn again, or otherwise return to their previous behavior. This slippage can result from a teacher or other person who is working with the child being too demanding; it is an indication that the child is feeling overwhelmed.

It's important to pay attention to these signs and intervene, says Madaule. The overwhelmed feeling and the attendant regression can have other sources, too. The child may simply be preparing for a new stage of development. Or it could be the result of a physical malady, such as an ear infection or allergies. Whatever the source, it is a sign that the child needs help, says Madaule. He tells parents to contact him if they see something like this for more than two weeks.

Those who have an autistic person in their life also need to understand a vital point about the brain, says Madaule. He notes that neuroscience is now saying what Dr. Tomatis, Madaule, and other clinicians have said for a long time: The brain keeps developing well beyond the first years of life but, in order to develop, the brain needs to be stimulated. Television does not qualify as stimulation; on the contrary, it increases the passivity of the brain. For this reason, Madaule advocates "pulling the plug on the TV. . . . Autistic kids can take a video and listen to it ten times in a day if you let them. That is not good for an autistic brain, and it's not good for your brain. If I was doing that to you, your brain would not think too much after a few months."

One of the problems with autism, he explains, is that the child doesn't know how to stimulate himself appropriately, as other children do, so he does not feed his brain. "After years of that, the brain is going to fall asleep. The brain needs food (which is why diet is very important), air (which is why oxygen and the quality of air is very important), and sensory stimuli to keep itself alive," says Maudale. Listening training provides the brain with the food it may be starving for, which is one of the reasons why its effects are so far reaching.

"Listening training is not a cure," concludes Madaule, "but we can significantly improve the communication problem of the autistic." This has ramifications for awareness, receptivity, self-control, and socialization, in addition to the obvious benefits for communication, learning, and language skills.

11 *Neural Therapy, Toxic Clearing, and Family Systems Therapy: The Levels of Healing*

While many people speak generally of the body-mind-spirit connection, Dietrich Klinghardt, M.D., Ph.D., based in Bellevue, Washington, has developed a detailed paradigm that explains that connection in terms of five levels of healing: the Physical Level, the Electromagnetic Level, the Mental Level, the Intuitive Level, and the Spiritual Level. Interferences or imbalances can occur at any of the five levels and travel upward or downward to other levels. Healing interventions can also be implemented at any of the levels, but unless upper-level imbalances are addressed, restoring balance at the lower levels will not produce long-lasting effects.

Clinically, Dr. Klinghardt has discovered that in the case of autism the first two levels—the Physical and the Electromagnetic—are typically involved. The fourth (Intuitive) level is also frequently implicated. Before we go into the levels in more detail, let's look at a case history that illustrates the relationship between autism and interferences at the first two levels of healing, and how the therapies Dr. Klinghardt uses to remove these interferences can ameliorate, and even reverse, severe autism.

Marcus: Heavy Metals, Vaccines, and Neural Interference

Marcus was six years old and severely developmentally delayed when his parents brought him to Dr. Klinghardt. He had been diagnosed with autism years before. He was withdrawn, did not engage in eye contact, did not talk aside from a few basic words (yes, no, Mom, Dad), and walked clumsily. When he was upset, he would smash his head against a wall, to the point of injury if not stopped. As a result, he wore a helmet most of the time. He was pale and would eat only white bread and sweets. To get him to eat any other foods, his parents had to resort to force feeding.

Marcus' development had been abnormal since birth. He rejected breast feeding, although he would take infant formula, cried all the time, and didn't relate or connect with either of his parents. At the age of six months, three days after his third major set of vaccines (his parents think these were MMR and DPT), his condition really deteriorated. He began to look very pale and unwell, and the head banging started.

His parents tried various behavioral approaches, which failed to produce improvement. In the year before consulting Dr. Klinghardt, Marcus received CranioSacral therapy regularly, which the parents felt had helped him quite a bit, particularly in the area of language. It was only after this intervention that he began to speak his few basic words.

See Also **For more about CranioSacral therapy, see chapter 9.**

Through autonomic response testing (ART), Dr. Klinghardt determined that Marcus had a condition known in the field of neural therapy as "blocked regulation." (See the sidebar for descriptions of the therapies used.) This refers to the "inability of the autonomic nervous system (ANS) to respond to any type of stimulus in an appropriate way," he explains.

The ANS controls the automatic processes of the body such as

About the Therapies and Techniques

Autonomic response testing (ART) is a system of testing developed by Dr. Klinghardt. It employs a variety of methods, including muscle response testing and arm length testing, among others, that measure changes in the autonomic nervous system. ART is used to identify distress in the body and determine optimum treatment. In general, a strong arm (or finger, depending on the kind of muscle testing) or an even arm length (in arm length testing) indicates that the system is not in distress. A weak muscle or uneven arm length indicates the presence of a factor that is causing stress to the client's organism.

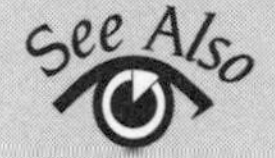

For more about muscle testing, see chapter 5.

Chelation is a therapy that removes heavy metals from the body, among other therapeutic functions. The substance *DMPS* (2,3-dimercaptopropane-1-sulfonate) is used as a chelating agent, which means that it binds with heavy metals, notably mercury, and is then excreted from the body. It can be administered orally, intravenously, or intramuscularly.

Neural therapy, developed by German physicians in 1925, employs the injection of local anesthetics such as lidocaine or procaine into specific sites in the body to clear interferences in the flow of electrical energy and restore proper nerve function. The interferences can be the result of a scar, other old injury, physical trauma, or dental conditions such as root-canalled or impacted teeth, all of which have their own energy fields that can disrupt the body's normal energy flow.

This disruption has far flung effects, and can manifest in seemingly unrelated conditions. "Any part of the body that has been traumatized or ill—no matter where it is located—can become an interference field which may cause disturbance anywhere in the body," states Dr. Klinghardt.[201]

Given that every cell relies on a system of electrical charges to function correctly, an interference in electrical energy can wreak havoc. In order to take in nutrients and eliminate wastes, the cell depends upon a regulated difference between the electrical charge inside and outside the cell, called the "membrane potential." When the membrane potential is skewed by an interference field, the cell's basic operations are compromised. The injection of anesthetics interrupts the electrical disturbance at the site of injection, restores proper nerve function, and restores the cellular membrane potential to its natural state, allowing cells to dump their accumulated toxins and begin to function normally again. The health benefits of returning the body's electrical flow to normal are as far reaching as the negative effects of disturbances in that flow.

Neural therapy injections may be into glands, acupuncture points, or ganglia (nerve bundles that are like relay stations for nerve impulses), as well as scars or sites of trauma.

respiration, heart rate, digestion, and response to stress. When the ANS is not responding appropriately, it usually means a high level of toxicity in the connective tissue and in the lymphatic system (the body's toxin filtering system), notes Dr. Klinghardt. Autonomic response training confirmed high mercury levels in Marcus' central nervous system (CNS). Composed of the spinal cord and brain, the CNS is integral to autonomic nervous function.

Marcus' mother had disclosed during the intake history that while she was pregnant with him, she had had eight old mercury amalgam fillings replaced with new mercury amalgams. The dental work lasted from week six to week twelve of the pregnancy. As noted in previous chapters, mercury from the mother, whether the source is dental fillings or fish in the diet, can pass to the infant via the placental blood supply.

To rid the body of the mercury and address the nervous system dysfunction, Dr. Klinghardt used chelation and neural therapy in combination. He gave a series of injections, containing a mixture of the chelator DMPS (see sidebar) and the anesthetic procaine. On each of four monthly visits, Marcus received an injection in the buttock along with what is known in neural therapy as a "crown of thorns." The latter is a ring of injections around the skull, and is typically used for head injuries.

Dr. Klinghardt chose this technique because of all the concussions Marcus had suffered over the years from banging his head against the wall. The injection mixture would treat the concussions while selectively driving the mercury from the brain. For further detoxification, Dr. Klinghardt started Marcus on an oral program. He took daily doses of the oral chelators alpha lipoic acid, chlorella, and cilantro, known to help pull heavy metals out of the body.

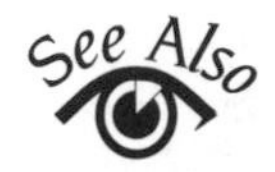

For more about oral chelation, see chapter 4.

Initial testing also revealed that Marcus had a condition called "neurogenic switching," a term used in both neurology and neural therapy. In neurogenic switching, the two hemispheres of the brain don't communicate with each other, a dysfunction other doctors have associated with autism. Numerous tests can identify this problem, but perhaps the most basic one is having the child turn his head one way and his eyes the other.

The autonomic nervous system of someone with neurogenic switching immediately goes into a stress state upon doing this, explains Dr. Klinghardt. The person breaks out in a sweat and the heart rate and blood pressure go up. Another indication of neurogenic switching is apparent in walking. If the person moves the same arm and leg together when stepping forward rather than the opposite arm and leg, which is normal, they may have this condition.

In Marcus' case, ART connected the neurogenic switching to the MMR vaccine. "The vaccine interfered with the communication between the two hemispheres of the brain," explains Dr. Klinghardt. "It is one of the things that we commonly see. We always test the vaccine when we see neurogenic switching." Like other doctors in this book, he uses the homeopathic MMR nosode to clear that vaccine. Marcus got one dose per month for six months.

For the first six weeks of treatment, all of Marcus' symptoms worsened, which Dr. Klinghardt expected, having seen this happen with many other children similar to Marcus. After six weeks, however, the mother reported that her son showed clear signs of getting better. Over the next two weeks, he spoke a complete sentence for the first time ever, began making occasional eye contact with both parents, and asked for solid food—meat, chicken, and fish—instead of his standard white bread and sweets. For the first time, he ate it on his own, without being forced.

At the end of five months of treatment, his mother rated him eighty percent better. He was speaking, relating to his parents, and no longer wore the helmet as he had stopped banging his head. He was also eating a good diet, high in protein and vegetables, and he was off grains and dairy.

Dr. Klinghardt agrees with the many practitioners who advocate taking autistic children off grains and dairy. In his experience, most do better on the gluten-free/casein-free diet. These substances have a morphine-like structure, he explains. "[W]hen autistic children lack the enzyme that breaks down the amino acid sequences in gluten completely, they absorb fragments that are identical to morphine. So they get that short morphine high from eating gluten." The same is true of casein. The morphine high from either narcotizes the child, making the brain sleepy.

He recommends cutting grain and dairy out gradually, however, because the withdrawal can be long and painful. It is "like getting a heroin addict off heroin." With autistic children, when you take them off grains and dairy cold turkey, they can experience some serious physiological detoxification symptoms, cautions Dr. Klinghardt, citing accelerated heart rate, temperature instabilities (from suddenly very cold to burning up), and even suddenly very high blood pressure. "We have to consider the physical addiction that needs to be dealt with gradually, not all at once."

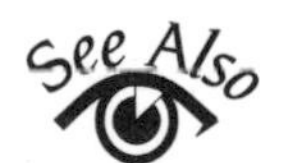

For more about gluten and casein, see chapter 2.

In Marcus' case, his mother reported that it was impossible to wean him from those foods in the first two months without enduring constant temper tantrums. By doing it gradually, she was able to get him off them by the end of five months.

After five months of treatment, Marcus turned seven and shortly afterwards started going to school for the first time. (This was only a year later than what would have been his normal starting time.) Although he was hyperactive and difficult at school, he could keep up with the academic tasks. His problems lay in relating to the other children and not being able to sit still. The teacher had to call the parents numerous times to come and get Marcus because she couldn't contain him.

At seven months into the treatment program, ART revealed another layer necessary for Marcus' healing. It showed that his umbilicus was what neural therapists call an "interference field," meaning "it was scarred and sending out abnormal electrical messages," states Dr. Klinghardt. This is not uncommon, he notes, as the belly button is the site of a physical trauma—the cutting of the umbilical cord. He injected the belly button with procaine and repeated the crown of thorns technique, again using the combination of procaine and DMPS.

Marcus' mother reported an amazing occurrence. The morning after the neural therapy, her son was completely well. "It was as if he had snapped into normal young boy behavior," Dr. Klinghardt recalls. "He was no longer in the category of hyperactive or any category of anything other than normal, and had total, normal development after that."

The last follow-up appointment Dr. Klinghardt had with Marcus was two years ago. Marcus was 12 years old by then and doing fine.

The Five Levels of Healing

As mentioned previously, Marcus' autism involved the first two levels in Dr. Klinghardt's paradigm of healing. The following section elucidates the five levels and identifies the therapeutic modalities that can remove interferences at each. Then we will look specifically at the causes and manifestation of interference at levels one, two, and four in autism.

The First Level: The Physical Body

The Physical Body includes all the functions on the physical plane, such as the structure and biochemistry of the body. Interference or imbalance at this level can result from an injury or anything that alters the structure: surgery, accidents, concussions, or dental work. "Surgery modulates the structure by creating adhesions...in the bones, the ligaments, changing the way things act on the structural level," says Dr. Klinghardt.

Imbalance at the first level can also result from anything that alters the biochemistry such as poor diet, too much or too little of a nutrient in the diet or in nutritional supplements, or taking the wrong supplements for one's particular biochemistry. Microorganisms such as bacteria or viruses can also change the biochemistry, as can parasites or worms. "They all take over the host to some degree and change the host behavior by modulating its biochemistry," Dr. Klinghardt explains.

"The whole world of toxicity belongs in the biochemistry department, too," he says. Toxic elements that can alter biochemistry include heavy metals, insecticides, pesticides, and all the other environmental chemicals. Interestingly, heavy metals operate on both the Physical Level and the next level of healing, the Electromagnetic Level. Due to their metallic nature, they can alter the biochemistry and also create electromagnetic disturbances.

All of these factors at the Physical Level—surgery, injury, dental work, nutritional imbalances, microorganisms, toxins—can play a role in producing symptoms of mental illness, according to Dr. Klinghardt.

The therapeutic modalities that function at this level are those that address biochemical or structural aspects, from drug and hormone therapies to herbal medicine and nutritional supplements, as well as mechanical therapies such as chiropractic.

The Second Level: The Electromagnetic Body

The Electromagnetic Body is the body's energetic field. Dr. Klinghardt explains it in terms of the traffic of information in the nervous system. "Eighty percent of the messages are going up to the brain [from the body], and twenty percent of the messages go down from the brain [to the body]. The nerve currents moving up and down generate a magnetic field that goes out into space, creating an electromagnetic field around the body that interacts with other fields." Acupuncture meridians (energy channels) and the chakra system are part of the Electromagnetic Body.

A chakra, which means 'wheel' in Sanskrit, is an energy vortex or center in the nonphysical counterpart (energy field) of the body. There are seven major chakras positioned roughly from the base of the spine, with points along the spine, to the crown of the head. As with acupuncture meridians, when chakras are blocked, the free flow of energy in the body's field is impeded.

Biophysical stress is a source of disturbance at this level. Biophysical stress is electromagnetic interference from devices that have their own electromagnetic fields, such as electric wall outlets, televisions, microwaves, cell phones, cell phone towers, power lines, and radio stations. These interfere with the electromagnetic system in the body. For example, if you sleep with your head near an electric outlet in the wall, the electromagnetic field from that outlet interferes with your own. An outlet may not even have to be involved. Simply sleeping with your head near a wall in which electric cables run can be sufficient to throw your field off. The brain's blood vessels typically contract in response to the man-made electromagnetic field, leading to decreased blood flow in the brain, says Dr. Klinghardt. A child may become hyperactive or develop a seizure disorder as a result of the electromagnetic interference and decreased blood flow.

Geopathic stress, or electromagnetic emission from the Earth, is another source of disturbance. Underground streams and fault lines are a source of these emissions. Again, proximity of your bed to one of these sources—for example, directly over a fault line—can throw your own electromagnetic field out of balance and produce a wide range of symptoms. Simply shifting the position of your bed in the room may remove the problem.

Interference at the second level can trickle down to the Physical Level. The constriction of the blood vessels in the brain in response to biophysical or geopathic stress results in the blood carrying less oxygen and nutrients to the brain. Nutritional deficiencies are a biochemical disturbance. If such deficiencies have their root at the Electromagnetic Level, however, it is important to know that you cannot fix them by taking supplements to correct the biochemistry, cautions Dr. Klinghardt.

For example, if an individual has a zinc deficiency, supplementing with zinc may correct the problem if it is merely a biochemical disturbance (a first-level issue). If the restriction of blood flow in the brain as a result of sleeping too close to an electrical outlet (a second-level issue) is behind the deficiency, taking zinc may seem to resolve the problem, but it will return when the person stops taking the supplement. Moving the bed away from the outlet will stop the electromagnetic interference and prevent the recurrence of a zinc deficiency.

Physical trauma or scars can also throw off the second level. "If a scar crosses an acupuncture meridian, it completely alters the energy flow in the system," observes Dr. Klinghardt. An infected tooth or a root canal can accomplish the same. Heavy metal toxicity, from mercury dental fillings and/or environmental metals in the air, water, and food supply, can block the entire electromagnetic system. "We know that the electrical activity in the autonomic ganglia really creates the chakras, and the ganglia can be disturbed by a lot of things, but toxicity in general is often responsible for throwing off the electromagnetic impulses," says Dr. Klinghardt. Vaccines can also do that.

The therapies that address this level of healing are those that correct the distortions of the body's electromagnetic field. Acupuncture and neural therapy are two strong modalities for this level. Neural therapy's injection of local anesthetic in the ganglion breaks up electromagnetic disturbance. You could call the local anesthetic "liquid electricity," says Dr. Klinghardt.

Another therapeutic modality that functions at the second level is Ayurvedic medicine (the traditional medicine of India). As it employs a combination of herbs and energetic interventions, it actually covers the first two levels of healing: the herbs work on the Physical Level, and the energetic aspect on the Electromagnetic Level.

The Third Level: The Mental Body

The third level is the Mental Level or the Mental Body, also known as the thought field. This is where your attitudes, beliefs, and early childhood experiences are. "This is the home of psychology," says Dr. Klinghardt. He explains that the Mental Body is outside the physical body, rather than housed in the brain. "We know now that memory and thinking, the mind, these are all phenomena outside the physical body. They're not happening in the brain as it was thought [previously]." The Mental Body is an energetic field.

Disturbances at this level come from traumatic experiences, beginning as early as conception. Early trauma or an unresolved conflict situation leaves faulty circuitry in the Mental Body, explains Dr. Klinghardt. For example, if at two years old, your parents divorced and your father was not allowed by law to see you, you may have formed the beliefs that your father didn't love you and that it was your fault your parents broke up because you are inherently bad. These damaging beliefs are faulty circuitry.

The brain replays traumatic experiences over and over, keeping constant stress signals running through the autonomic nervous system. This disturbance trickles down into the Electromagnetic Level of healing, triggering the constriction of blood vessels, and in turn, trickling down to the biochemical level in the form of nutritional deficiencies.

It may look like a biochemical disturbance, says Dr. Klinghardt, but the cause is much higher up. "Again, this is a situation you cannot lastingly fix by giving someone supplements or neural therapy or acupuncture." You have to address the third-level interference, the problem in the Mental Body.

Among the therapeutic modalities that work at this level are psychotherapy, hypnotherapy, homeopathy, and applied psychoneurobiology (APN), which was developed by Dr. Klinghardt. Employing his muscle testing method as a guide, APN uses stress signals in the autonomic nervous system to communicate with a patient's unconscious mind. "You can establish a code with the unconscious mind for 'yes' and 'no' in answer to questions," he explains. "The code is the strength or the weakness of a test muscle."

APN can lead the way to the beliefs that underlie the chronic illness and exchange those beliefs with ones that promote balance in the Mental Body. This can produce dramatic shifts in the health of the person, notes Dr. Klinghardt.

Mental disease isn't necessarily a function of disturbance in the Mental Body. "People might think, 'These are called mental diseases, therefore they must be on the Mental Body.' It has nothing to do with that. Mental disease is primarily a phenomenon on the Physical Body, at the lowest level, but the cause can be on any of the five levels." Again, the source level must be addressed or lasting resolution will not be achieved.

In terms of autism, the causes are not typically on the Mental Level, according to Dr. Klinghardt. "In my experience, it rarely is a psychological experience in the household that's causing autism. Or let's put it this way, by working with families on the psychological issues, I've rarely seen an autistic child get well." By the way, the now debunked "refrigerator mother" theory of autism would have been on this level.

The Fourth Level: The Intuitive Body

The fourth level is the Intuitive Body. Some people call it the Dream Body. Experience on this level includes dream states, trance states, and ecstasy, as well as states with a negative association such as nightmares, possession, and curses. The Intuitive Body is what Jung called the collective unconscious. "On the fourth level, humans are deeply connected with each other and also with all animals, rocks, stones, and the planet," says Dr. Klinghardt.

The fourth level is the home of shamanism. Other healers who can work at this level to remove interference are those who practice transpersonal psychology. Stated simply, transpersonal refers to an acknowledgment of the phenomena of the fourth level, "the dimension where a person is affected deeply in themselves by something that isn't of themselves, that is of somebody else. Transpersonal psychology is really a cover-up term for modern shamanism," observes Dr. Klinghardt.

For healing of the Intuitive Body, Dr. Klinghardt uses what is known as systemic family therapy, or family systems therapy. It addresses interference that comes from a previous generation in the family. In this type of interference, he says, "the cause and effect are separated by several generations. It goes over time and over space." Rather than a genetic inheritance of a physical weakness, it is an energetic legacy of an injustice with which the family never dealt.

"A member of the family two, three, or four generations later will atone for that injustice in their life without ever knowing who the person was who did something," explains Dr. Klinghardt. For example, a woman murders her husband and is never found out. She marries again and lives a long life. Three generations later, one of her great-grandchildren is born. To atone for the murder, the child self-sacrifices. He may develop brain cancer when he is three years old. He may be murdered, may be abused. As a teenager, he may start taking drugs and commit slow suicide that way.

"It's a form of self-punishment that anybody can see on the outside, but nobody understands what's wrong with this child—he had loving parents, good nutrition, went to a good school, and look what he's doing now, he's on drugs. But if you look back two or three generations, you'll see exactly why this child is self-sacrificing." Dr. Klinghardt notes that mental illness is "very, very often an outcome on the systemic level."

Systemic family therapy involves tracing the origins of current illness back to a previous generation. For the discovery process, Dr. Klinghardt uses the systemic family therapy developed by German psychoanalyst Bert Hellinger. Sometimes an event is known in a family, sometimes it is not. By questioning a client, Dr. Klinghardt is usually able to discover an event from a previous generation that is a likely source of interference for the client's current troubles. If no one knew about a certain event, such as the murder in the example above, there are usually clues in a family that point to those people as a possible source.

For the therapy, the client or a close relative chooses audience members to represent the people in question. In our example, they would be the great-grandmother, great-grandfather, and the new husband. These people come together on a stage or central area. They are not told the story, even when the story is known.

"They just go up there not knowing anything, and suddenly feel all these feelings and have all these thoughts come up. . . . Very quickly, within a minute or two, they start feeling like the real people in life have felt, or are feeling in their death now, and start interacting with each other in bizarre ways," says Dr. Klinghardt.

The client typically does not participate, but simply observes. "The therapist does careful therapeutic interventions, but there's very little needed usually." The person put up for the murdered husband stands there, with no idea of what happened in the past, but then he falls to the floor. When someone asks, "What happened to you?" he answers, "I've been murdered." It just comes out of his mouth. Then the therapist asks if he wants to say anything to any of the other people. He speaks to his wife and it becomes clear that she was the one who murdered him. They speak back and forth, and "very quickly, there's deep healing that happens between the two," states Dr. Klinghardt. "Usually we relive the pain and the truth that was there . . . It's very, very dramatic . . . Then the therapist does some therapeutic intervention with those representatives."

With removal of the interference that was transmitted down the generations, the client's condition is resolved, although the trickle-down effect to the lower levels of healing may need to be addressed. Often, however, healing at the higher level is sufficient. With balance restored at that level, the other levels are then able to correct themselves.

Dr. Klinghardt likens family systems therapy to shamanic work in Africa, in which healing often has to be done from a distance through a representative because of the impracticability of having a sick child, for example, travel two hundred miles from the village to see the medicine man. The representative holds a piece of clothing or hair from that child, and the shaman does the healing work on the stranger. "There's a magical effect, broadcast back to the child," says Dr. Klinghardt. "The child gets well. It's the same principle [with family systems therapy]. We call it surrogate healing." He adds that systemic family therapy has become very popular in Europe in the last two years, while it is still relatively new in the United States.

Dr. Klinghardt has developed a variation of this technique that enables the work to happen with just a practitioner and the patient. He accomplishes the same end without representatives of the antecedents, using ART to pinpoint what happened and engage in the dialogues that arise in this work. He gives the example of a forty-five-year-old woman who had lived daily with asthma since she was two years old.

Through ART muscle testing, in a kind of process of elimination, Dr. Klinghardt learned that physical causes were not the source of the asthma and that it had to do with exclusion of some kind in a previous generation. Further exploration revealed that this woman's mother had lost a younger sibling when *she* was two years old. In this case, the woman knew of the event, but that was all she knew. ART confirmed the connection between this buried death and the asthma. Dr. Klinghardt stopped the session at this point, instructing his client to find out what she could about this family occurrence and then come back.

The woman's mother was still alive and told her that the baby died shortly after birth, was buried behind the house without a gravestone or other marker on the site, and was never mentioned again in the family. Everyone knew where the child was buried, but there was an unspoken agreement never to speak of her. Not only that, but the next child born was given the same name, as if the one who had died had never existed.

"This was a violation of a principle of what we know from systemic family therapy, which is that each member that's born into a family has the same and equal right to belong to the family." Exclusion, even in memory, is a form of injustice, and creates interference energy that is transmitted through the generations. Exclusion of a family member in the past is frequently the source of disturbance at the intuitive level, according to Dr. Klinghardt.

The client came back for the second session, and Dr. Klinghardt put her into a light trance state. "In that trance state she was able to contact that being, the dead sibling, and say to her, 'I remember you now, I bring you back into my family, I give you a place in my heart, I will never forget you.' Then she cried, and it was a very transformative experience." He observes that this process required very little guidance from him and took only about 20 minutes.

During the session, the woman made a commitment to go back to the house where the child was buried—it was still a family property—and put a gravestone on her grave. After the session, the woman's asthma was clearly better. She rated it at 50 to 60 percent better, and reported later that it stayed that way. "It took her about three months to put up the gravestone, and she said the day after she set up the gravestone for that child, her asthma disappeared completely," relates Dr. Klinghardt. That was eight years ago and the asthma has not returned.

Dr. Klinghardt and others who practice family systems therapy have seen similar connections in cases of mental illness. Chronic depression, schizophrenia, addiction, hyperactivity in children, aggressive behavior, and autism can all lead back to systemic family issues.

The Fifth Level: The Spiritual

The fifth level is the direct relationship of the patient with God, or whatever name you choose for the divine spirit. This level requires self-healing when there is separation or interference in that connection. "True prayer, true meditation, work on this level as ways of getting there, but it's a level where there is no possibility of interaction between the healer and the patient," states Dr. Klinghardt. "I always say, if anybody tries to be helpful on this level, run as fast as you can." He notes that gurus (spiritual teachers) belong on the fourth level and have a valuable place there, but have no business on the fifth level. If they trespass into that level, they are putting themselves where God should be, says Dr. Klinghardt. "It's very dangerous."

The Spiritual Level is not typically implicated in autism.

Operating Principles of the Healing Levels

The levels affect each other differently, depending on whether the influence is traveling upward or downward. A trauma or successful therapeutic intervention at the higher levels has a rapid and deeply penetrating effect on the lower levels, says Dr.

Klinghardt. This means that both the cause and the cure at the upper levels spread downward quickly. For example, if a systemic family issue is strongly present at the fourth level, the Intuitive Level, it will have profound effects on the first three levels. Similarly, resolving that issue can produce rapid changes in the Physical, Electromagnetic, and Mental Bodies.

The factors that contribute to autism at the physical level are those related to biochemistry and structure. Heavy metal toxicity is high on this list. "We know that the growing nervous system of a fetus is highly vulnerable to exposure to toxic metals," states Dr. Klinghardt. "They come through the mother to the placenta, and also through the mother's milk."

At the same time, a trauma or therapeutic intervention at the lower levels has a very slow and little penetrating effect upwards. When you get a physical injury (the first level), for instance, it will gradually change your electromagnetic field (the second level), altering the energy flow in your body. It's a slow process, however. "If you want to heal an injury on the second level, let's say you have a chakra that's blocked, you can do that by giving herbs and vitamins—biochemical interventions—but it will take years," says Dr. Klinghardt. But if you do an intervention on the third or fourth level, it can correct the blocked chakra on the second level immediately, within seconds or minutes, he notes.

Autism and the Healing Levels

As noted previously, the levels most often involved in autism are the first, second, and fourth levels—the Physical, Electromagnetic, and Intuitive Bodies.

Autism and the First Level

The factors that contribute to autism at the Physical Level are those related to biochemistry and structure. Heavy metal toxicity is high on this list. "We know that the growing nervous system of a fetus is highly vulnerable to exposure to toxic metals," states Dr. Klinghardt. "They come through the mother to the placenta, and also through the mother's milk. Basically, the pregnant mother uses the growing fetus as a garbage can for her unresolved stuff." This "stuff" includes dioxin, formaldehyde, and other toxins in addition to heavy metals such as mercury.

Children who have had significant heavy metal exposure in the womb are already "on the edge" due to this toxic overload when they are born. When they are hit with vaccines containing more mercury, that's "the second strike," says Dr. Klinghardt. Autism can ensue. Like others in this book, he cautions against focusing exclusively on the heavy metal issue in vaccines. "I have a feeling that by focusing on the heavy metals that used to be used in the vaccine, the government is trying to distract people from the fact that the vaccines themselves are dangerous."

Even without heavy metal preservatives, vaccines are another predominant first-level factor in autism. Like many physicians and other health-care practitioners, Dr. Klinghardt has seen numerous children with autism that was linked to the aftermath of vaccinations. In his experience, MMR is the most common culprit, but the hepatitis B and pertussis vaccines have been instrumental in a number of cases as well. Pertussis used to figure more prominently in the autism cases he saw, but since the vaccine was changed a couple of years ago to a milder version, it's not as damaging, or not as frequently damaging, as it used to be, he reports.

Autonomic Response Testing can identify the connection between an individual child's autism and specific vaccines. For example, muscle testing indicators of the illness may "resonate" with the hepatitis B vaccine, which means there is a strong "yes" from the test muscle that the autism is connected to that particular vaccine. There is often a multiple vaccine connection, Dr. Klinghardt notes, supporting the data that indicate that there is a synergetic effect between the vaccines. "The more vaccines, the more chance of developing autism," he states.

Like the heavy metals, the vaccine viruses impair various biochemical systems, including the enzyme system. "On the most superficial level, people develop a deep disturbance in their fatty acid metabolism. We know that for sure," says Dr. Klinghardt. Vaccines also change the bowel flora in favor of pathogenic microorganisms, another first-level issue. "The situation in the bowel sets the child up for allergies, eczema, and asthma. The four A's, we call them: autism, allergies, asthma, and atopic dermatitis (allergic skin reactions or skin illnesses)." He often sees these other three A's in autistic children.

In terms of the immune system, the effects of the vaccines go far beyond short-term weakened immunity, says Dr. Klinghardt. To understand this, we need to look at two types of immunity: humoral immune response and cell-mediated immune response. The first involves the production of antibodies in the blood in response to the presence of foreign antigens (protein markers); immunity or hypersensitivity can result from this response. The second involves the production of important immune "workers" (T cells) that migrate around the body and capture microorganisms. The latter system is not mature until the end of the first two years of life.

"What you do with the vaccine is stimulate the hell out of the humoral immune system at the expense of the cellular immune system," explains Dr. Klinghardt. "That means the cellular immune system is impaired, it grows up crippled, never achieving full maturity, competence, and intelligence. The secondary damage from the vaccines is because of the immaturity of the cellular immune system. The child, and later the adult, will be prone to developing allergies or hidden infections." By postponing the onset of the first vaccines until after the child is 24 months old, the secondary damage could be greatly reduced and the problem of an undeveloped immune system avoided.

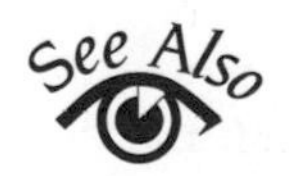

For more about vaccines and the two aspects of immunity, see chapter 7.

The structural factors involved in autism on the Physical Level are those explained by Dr. Lavine in chapter 8: the distortions and compressions of the skull that result from birth, particularly in the epidural/Pitocin births that are so common in modern obstetrics. These structural damages have biochemical effects throughout the body and also produce electromagnetic interferences, thus operating directly on both the first and second levels.

Another important electromagnetic issue to consider with autistic children is whether they are sleeping with their heads near a wall with electric cables in it. This is not good for any children, but it is particularly dangerous for those with autism. "Heavy metals work like microantennae, little antennas inside the brain," says Dr. Klinghardt.

As Dr. Lavine noted, the function of neurotransmitters in the brain, another biochemical issue, is compromised by compression of the skull. In addition, biochemical problems associated with autism, such as the fatty acid disturbances, create a rigidity in the skull bones, notes Dr. Klinghardt. "Then the rigidity in the skull bones worsens the autism, and the autism worsens the rigidity. It's a vicious cycle."

Chelation to rid the body of the heavy metals, other detoxification protocols, homeopathic nosodes to clear the vaccines, and nutritional and herbal supplements to help restore deficient biochemistry and rebalance intestinal flora are all therapeutic interventions for first-level factors in autism. CranioSacral therapy works on both the first and second levels of healing, correcting the structural interferences of birth-related traumas and the attendant electromagnetic interferences. It also breaks the vicious cycle of biochemical and structural disturbances interacting to worsen autism.

Autism and the Second Level

As stated previously, physical trauma can throw off the electromagnetic field of the body, the second level. The cranial distortions and compressions caused by birth fall into this category and should not be overlooked as a source of electromagnetic interference in autism.

With the brain and spinal cord comprising the central nervous system, disturbance in this arena has obvious electromagnetic implications for the entire body. As noted above, CranioSacral therapy operates on both a physical and electromagnetic level. "A good CranioSacral therapist uses the electric field of his hand to initiate a lot of the healing that happens from the technique," says Dr. Klinghardt.

Scars, particularly the umbilicus, are another significant second-level issue in autism, as was the case with Marcus. In Dr. Klinghardt's view, the belly button is actually a scar, formed when the cord shrivels up after being cut. As with any scar, it can interfere with the energy flow in the body. Neural therapy is the solution here. "I had at least one case in which the autism was gone within a few weeks after an injection. It was a single intervention on the second level that cured the autism." Dr. Klinghardt has also reversed seizure problems and several cases of childhood epilepsy by injecting the umbilicus.

Another important electromagnetic issue to consider with autistic children is whether they are sleeping with their heads near a wall with electric cables in it. This is not good for any children, but it is particularly dangerous for those with autism. "Heavy metals work like microantennae, little antennas inside the brain," says Dr. Klinghardt.

"When you put a head of a child that's heavy metal toxic against a wall with an electric cable in it, then that electric field from the wall has a severely damaging effect on the development of the brain." He had a number of autism cases that improved significantly with a combination of heavy metal detoxification and moving the bed away from the wall. He advises placing the bed so any body part of the person sleeping in it is at least two feet away from the wall.

Autism and the Fourth Level

While the systemic family issues of the fourth level were not involved in Marcus's case, they are another factor to consider in approaching the treatment of autism. The range of specific issues that can be the source is vast, but it usually involves a family member who was excluded in a previous generation, like the dead child in the case of the woman with asthma. When the other family members don't go through the deep process of grieving the excluded one, whether the exclusion results from separation, death, alienation, or ostracism, the psychic interference of that exclusion is passed on.

While the most potent healing happens at the highest origin of the problem, autism is often multicausal, with distinct problems that arose at each level in addition to the problems created by the penetration of interference from above and below. For that reason, Dr. Klinghardt feels it is best to address all three levels: the Physical, the Electromagnetic, and the Intuitive.

Another common systemic factor involves identification with victims of a forebear. "I've found a class of autism in children of Vietnam vets," observes Dr. Klinghardt. These veterans carried a lot of guilt at having killed in a war they didn't regard as a "good war." The autistic children deeply identified with their father's victims, on a completely unconscious level, of course. "They lived as if they had been poisoned by Agent Orange or as if they had been shell-shocked by something—violence."

The healing comes when the father deeply grieves the violence he had to commit and perhaps what he didn't do as well—stop, refuse, intervene, protect. "When he honestly and deeply grieves and bows to those victims, that's when suddenly, the autistic child snaps out of it, sometimes overnight. The lights go on, and you have a normal child," says Dr. Klinghardt, adding, "This is something that unless you've seen it, you won't believe it. Nobody who reads this will believe it either." He has seen it happen numerous times, and with a similar issue in Germany as well.

"We had a cluster of that offspring of the Holocaust perpetrator generation," says Dr. Klinghardt, who is German. Again, the children deeply identified with the victims, and reenacted victimhood through their illnesses. In this case, it was not the children of the perpetrators, but the grandchildren. The systemic family issue skipped a generation and affected a cluster of children. In that way, it was a systemic issue of both family and culture. In Germany, in the first generation of Holocaust offspring, autism wasn't common, but now in the second generation, it's very common, according to Dr. Klinghardt.

You might respond that the rise in incidence could be related to increased use of vaccines. But again, "when the healing work is done, when the parents bow to the victims, and instigate a deep healing, the autism goes away. This is without any medical intervention." It provides a clear illustration of the fourth level in operation.

This does not mean there are not interferences on the lower levels in cases of autism, however. In fact, it's very uncommon for there not to be, says Dr. Klinghardt, given the way the levels work, with rapid penetration of the upper into the lower. When the fourth level penetrates through to the third level, neurotic behavior follows. When penetration reaches the second level, the result is odd phenomena in the nervous system, the acupuncture system, and the chakras. When it arrives at the first level, they get a "completely wacky biochemistry," he explains. Again, healing the biochemistry is not going to fix the problem when the source is at the fourth level.

A *Cascade of* Health

If you address the source and remove the interference at the fourth level, the therapeutic intervention cascades downward as rapidly as the interference did, and the lower levels may correct without further remediation. This is true of vaccine disturbance as well. Dr. Klinghardt finds he often doesn't have to deal with clearing the vaccines after correcting a problem at the fourth level.

While the most potent healing happens at the highest origin of the problem, autism is often multicausal, with distinct problems that arose at each level in addition to the problems created by the penetration of interference from above and below. For that reason, Dr. Klinghardt feels it is best to address all three levels: the Physical, the Electromagnetic, and the Intuitive.

In terms of remedial therapies such as speech therapy and sensory integration to help the child catch up with the development delayed by autism, Dr. Klinghardt has found that many of the children he has cleared of interferences catch up without such interventions. These therapies, however, "make the landing softer and faster," he says. They speed up the process and soften social integration and other aspects of the environment with which the child is newly dealing.

In sharp contrast to the gloomy prognosis many parents receive from their doctors when they are told their child is autistic, Dr. Klinghardt says, "The wonderful thing about autism is that it is to a large degree reversible even in a fairly progressed state."

Conclusion

What is the message of autism? What can we as individuals and a human community learn from what is now an epidemic disorder among us? I ask these questions because I believe that nothing is accidental, that everything that happens contains information for us.

Obviously, there is no one answer to these questions, and the answers may be different for everyone. In addition to the individual knowledge and rich experience that parents gain from living with a child with autism, perhaps there are certain messages that are common to us all.

Some of the lessons for us in this epidemic of autism may be: Attend to the environmental onslaught under which we are living and do something to help clean up our planet; do not accept medical practices without question, even when they are widely used; take responsibility for our own and our children's health instead of turning that responsibility over to a physician; don't accept a medical diagnosis as a dead end or even a definition of a health condition; and come together to address what is now a widespread community problem rather than infrequent isolated instances of a disorder.

Attend to the environmental onslaught under which we are living and do something to help clean up our planet.

Perhaps the epidemic of autism is another canary in the mine for the human race, putting us on alert that our environment is unhealthy, and further health consequences will follow if we don't do something about cleaning up our air, water, soil, and food supply. As discussed in chapter 2, environmental toxins may contribute to creating a weakened system that leaves a susceptible child vulnerable to developing autism. When other factors, such as vaccines, are introduced, they may tip the balance into overload, and neurological disturbances will ensue. By reducing, or preferably ending, the release of more toxins into our environment, and implementing policies and practices to clean up those that are already there, we take steps toward preventing the vulnerability of toxic overload in our children. Their health, and ours, can only benefit.

Do not accept medical practices without question, even when they are widely used.

Sometimes illness serves to open our eyes to what we blindly accept. For many of us, it took an illness before we began to question medical authority. There is ample evidence that doctors are not always right, and medical practices move in and out of favor. What is widely dispensed in one era is debunked in another. The use of prescription drugs as the solution to health problems is one current medical approach that needs to be questioned. Conventional medications mask symptoms and in most cases do not address the underlying causes of an illness. Drugs as the solution for autism are particularly suspect. As this book has shown, autism involves many contributing factors that can be systematically treated and eliminated. To fail to identify what is happening in the child's body and to offer behavior-controlling drugs as the only solution borders on the criminal.

Childhood immunizations are another medical practice that should not be accepted without question. As delineated in chapter 3, there is serious evidence to suggest that our current vaccination policies are detrimental to the health of our children and need to be reconsidered. Further research is essential and, given that vaccines may be a contributing factor in the development of autism, the policies should be amended to err on the side of safety until studies achieve conclusive results.

In the meantime, parents need to know that there are alternatives to proceeding along the recommended vaccination path.

Eliminating at-birth vaccinations, cutting down on the number of vaccines administered at one time, giving certain vaccines when the child is older, and using only vaccines that do not contain heavy metals are all ways to modify the vaccination protocol. Using homeopathy as an alternative to vaccines or to treat childhood illnesses as they arise is a means of avoiding the conventional protocol altogether.

The message is: Investigate for yourself.

Take responsibility for our own and our children's health instead of turning that responsibility over to a physician.

Illness can also teach us that we are ultimately responsible for our own health, and for that of our children. We need to take control of the healing process rather than expecting doctors to run the show for us. No one knows a child as well as the parents do, so it's important for the parents to be the ones who make the decisions and choose the direction treatment will take. This does not mean not seeking doctors' expert advice, but parents need to regard that advice as information to be considered along with other information they have gathered for the purpose of putting together a treatment program that will be best for their particular child. As this book has established, a multimodal approach to autism produces the best results.

Yes, it's a lot more work to approach health in this way, but the process is empowering and the outcome so much better.

Don't accept a medical diagnosis as a dead end or even a definition of a health condition.

The conventional prognosis for autism could be regarded as a dead end but, as this book has revealed, that is far from the reality. As illustrated by the case studies herein, many autistic children completely recover or significantly improve when the underlying factors in their individual conditions are removed or corrected. The concept of underlying factors relates to the second aspect of this lesson: the definition of a health condition. The label of autism provides no information about the factors that combined in a particular child to produce the disorder. To determine the medical treatment for a child with autism it is necessary to look beyond the diagnosis.

Again, it is necessary to identify the imbalances and deficiencies in the individual child's system. When approached in this way, treatment can be more systematic, comprehensive, and hopeful because the chances of success are greater. Moving beyond the diagnosis and definition of autism and considering the individual opens new vistas for treatment and poses the possibility of a healthy future.

Come together to address what is now a widespread community problem rather than infrequent isolated instances of a disorder.

Autism used to be a rarity but that is no longer the case. With an incidence of 1 in 150 in some places in the United States, parents with an autistic child are truly no longer alone. Support is both good for the health, as research has shown, and a necessary aspect of bringing an end to this epidemic. With the state of the environment and the existence of global medical policies, health is no longer an individual issue. Perhaps the ultimate message of the epidemic of autism is that we belong to a global community that needs to take responsibility for the health of all of its members.

Appendix A
Professional Degrees and Titles

C.M.P.	Certified Massage Practitioner
D.C.	Doctor of Chiropractic
D.Ht.	Diplomate in Homeotherapeutics
Di.Hom.	Diplomate in Homeopathy
D.O.	Doctor of Osteopathy
D.T.M.&H.	Diploma in Tropical Medicine and Health
H.M.D.	Homeopathic Medical Doctor
L.Ac.	Licensed Acupuncturist
L.Ps.	Licensié en Psychologie (French psychology degree)
M.P.H.	Masters in Public Health
M.S.W.	Masters in Social Work
N.M.D	Doctor of Naturopathic Medicine
N.D.	Doctor of Naturopathy
O.M.D.	Oriental Medical Doctor
R.M.T.	Registered Massage Therapist

Appendix B
Resources

Practitioners in this book

Richard E. Hiltner, M.D., D. Ht.
169 East El Roblar Drive
Ojai, CA 93023
Tel: (805) 646-1495
E-mail: rhiltner@pol.net
Specializes in family medicine, homeopathy, acupuncture, and traditional Chinese medicine

Dietrich Klinghardt, M.D., Ph.D.
1200 112th Avenue NE, Suite A100
Bellevue, WA 98004
Tel: (425) 688-8818
Specializes in neural therapy, applied psychoneurobiology, and family systems therapy to address the transgenerational energy legacies at the root of illness

Carola M. Lage-Roy, Naturopath-Homoeopath (Heilpraktikerin Homoeopathie)
2421 Summerhill Drive
Encinitas, CA 92024
Tel: (760) 943-7697 or 943-8885

In Germany:
Breite 2
82418 Murnau Germany
Tel: 001-49-8841-4455
Fax: 001-49-8841-4298
E-mail: homoeopathy@ravi-roy.de (note the European spelling of homoeopathy)
Web site: www.ravi-roy.de

In addition to their clinic, Lage-Roy and her husband, Ravi Roy, run Lage & Roy Publishing Company and have written 28 books on homoeopathy, including *Homoeopathic Guide—Vaccination Damage, Homoeopathic Guide—Infectious Diseases of Children, The Homoeopathic Family Home-Care,* and *Bioweapons and Homoeopathy.*

They also run the Ravi Roy Teaching and Research Institute for Homoeopathy and offer a correspondence course in homoeopathy.

Lawrence Lavine, D.O., M.P.H., D.T.M.&H.
9424 Veterans Drive SW
Tacoma, WA 98498
Tel: (253) 589-4625
E-mail: llavine@attglobal.net

Practice focuses on cranial osteopathy, osteopathic manipulative medicine, NAET, injury reversal, and the interaction of injuries and allergies. Dr. Lavine also has a special focus on autism using an integrative approach of osteopathy, NAET, nutrition, mercury detoxification, and intense rehabilitation.

Paul Madaule, L.Ps.
The Listening Centre
599 Markham Street
Toronto, Ontario M6G 2L7 Canada
Tel: (416) 588-4136
E-mail: listen@idirect.com
Website: www.listeningcentre.com

The Listening Centre is the first clinic in North America

using the Tomatis Method of listening training; providing remedial intervention for auditory processing disorders, attentional problems, learning disabilities, language delays, and communication problems as in autistic spectrum disorders. Paul Madaule, a French-trained psychologist, is the author of *When Listening Comes Alive: A Guide to Effective Learning and Communication.*

Devi S. Nambudripad, M.D., D.C., L.Ac., Ph.D.
Pain Clinic
6714 Beach Boulevard
[Nambudripad Allergy Research Foundation
6732 Beach Boulevard]
Buena Park, CA 90621
Tel: (714) 523-8900

The Pain Clinic treats various pain and allergy disorders using NAET (Nambudripad's Allergy Elimination Techniques), acupuncture, and chiropractic. The Allergy Research Foundation is a nonprofit organization devoted to conducting clinical trials and studies on NAET and educating the public and professionals alike. Dr. Nambudripad is the author of numerous books, including *Say Good-Bye to Allergy-Related Autism.*

Maile Pouls, Ph.D.
Health Enhancement Center
517 Liberty Street
Santa Cruz, CA 95060
Tel: (831) 423-7554
E-mail: drpouls@cruzio.com
Website: www.yournutrition.com

Clinical nutritionist specializing in Targeted Therapeutic Nutrition (including Special Needs Children's Nutritional Programs), an individualized treatment program based on nutritional, dietary, and symptom history and the results of 24-hour urinalysis and other body chemistry and toxic element panels (as needed); treatment focuses on reversing a condition by supporting the specific body systems and organs involved, correcting nutritional deficiencies, rebalancing body chemistry, and detoxifying the colon, liver, and lymphatic system. Dr. Pouls conducts appointments by phone as well as in person, so is available to clients in any location.

Judyth Reichenberg-Ullman, N.D., M.S.W.
The Northwest Center for Homeopathic Medicine
131 Third Avenue North
Edmonds, WA 98020
Tel: (425) 774-5599
Websites: www.healthyhomeopathy.com and
www.ritalinfreekids.com

In practice with her husband, Robert Ullman, Dr. Reichenberg-Ullman is a licensed naturopathic physician board-certified in homeopathy. She has been practicing for 18 years and is the author/co-author of six books on homeopathic medicine, including *Ritalin-Free Kids, Prozac-Free,* and *Whole Woman Homeopathy.*

Bernard Rimland, Ph.D.
Autism Research Institute (ARI)
4182 Adams Avenue
San Diego, CA 92116
Fax: (619) 563-6840
Website: www.autismresearchinstitute.com

Dr. Rimland is a research psychologist and director of ARI, a nonprofit organization dedicated to conducting and facilitating research on the cause, prevention, and treatment of autism and similar conditions. The Autism Research Institute, which publishes the *Autism Research Review International,* is also an excellent source of information about autism and serves as an important resource for parents and others seeking to know more about the disorder.

Zannah Steiner, C.M.P., R.M.T.
Soma Therapy Centre
2607 West 16th Avenue
Vancouver, BC V6K 3C2 Canada
Tel: (604) 731-7883

E-mail: soma@intouch.bc.ca
Website: www.somatherapy.info

The Centre offers a range of Soma (body) therapies, particularly utilizing CranioSacral therapy, Visceral Manipulation, and SomatoEmotional Release to address the root causes of a disorder. Other therapies include acupuncture, chiropractic, psychological counseling, massage, and hydrotherapy. Among the conditions commonly treated are autism, developmental delays, ADD, immune deficiencies, paralysis, depression, chronic fatigue, chronic pain, and addictions.

William J. Walsh, Ph.D.
Health Research Institute and Pfeiffer Treatment Center
1804 Centre Point Circle
Naperville, IL 60563
Tel: (630) 505-0300
E-mail: info@hriptc.org
Website: www.hriptc.org

Chief scientist/biochemical researcher at HRIPTC, a non-profit organization based in Illinois, with services in Minnesota, Maryland, Arizona, and California; outpatient clinic with collaboration between medical doctors, biochemists, and nutritionists, offering individualized nutrient therapy for autism, ADD, depression, bipolar disorder, schizophrenia, and other conditions.

Autism Organizations and Information Sources

Autism Network for Dietary Intervention (ANDI)
P.O. Box 17711
Rochester, NY 14617-0711
Fax: (609) 737-8453
Website: www.autismndi.com

Autism Research Institute (ARI)
4182 Adams Avenue
San Diego, CA 92116
Fax: (619) 563-6840

Website: www.autismresearchinstitute.com
DAN! (Defeat Autism Now) is a project of ARI
ARI also publishes the *Autism Research Review International.*

Autism Society of America
7910 Woodmont Avenue, Suite 300
Bethesda, MD 20814-3015
Phone: (800) 3AUTISM or (301)-657-0881
Website: www. autism-society.org

This is a mainstream organization that does not offer much in the way of alternative information.

Cure Autism Now (CAN)
5455 Wilshire Boulevard, Suite 715
Los Angeles, CA 90036
Phone: (888) 8AUTISM or (323) 549-0500
E-mail: email@cureautismnow.org
Website: www.cureautismnow.org

In addition to these websites, the following are good sources of information on autism and autism-related subjects:

Allergy induced Autism: www.kessick.demon.co.uk/aia.htm
Autism sites listing/links: www.autism.com
Illinois Vaccine Awareness Coalition (IVAC): www.vaccineawareness.org
Dr. Joseph Mercola: www.mercola.com (great research source on mercury and other topics)
National Vaccine Information Center (NVIC): www.909shot.com
PROVE (Parents Requesting Open Vaccine Education): www.vaccineinfo.net
Dr. Tinus Smits: www.tinussmits.com (great research source on vaccines, homeopathy, and other topics)

Recommended Reading

Baker, Sidney M., M.D., and Jon Pangborn, Ph.D. *Biomedical Assessment Options for Children with Autism and Related Problems.* A Consensus Report of the Defeat Autism Now! (DAN!) Conference, Dallas, Texas, January 1995. San Diego, California: Autism Research Institute, 1999. (Available from the Autism Research Institute)

Frith, Uta. *Autism: Explaining the Enigma.* Cambridge, Massachusetts: Blackwell, 1989.

Grandin, Temple, and Margaret M. Scariano. *Emergence: Labeled Autistic.* New York: Warner Books, 1996.

Madaule, Paul. *When Listening Comes Alive: A Guide to Effective Learning and Communication.* Norval, Ontario: Moulin, 1994.

Nambudripad, Devi S., D.C., L.Ac., R.N., Ph.D. *Say Goodbye to Allergy-Related Autism.* Buena Park, California: Delta Publishing, 1999.

Park, Clara Claiborne. *The Siege: A Family's Journey into the World of an Autistic Child.* New York: Little, Brown & Co., 1995.

Reichenberg-Ullman, Judyth, N.D., M.S.W., and Robert Ullman, N.D. *Ritalin-Free Kids: Safe and Effective Homeopathic Medicine for ADHD, and Other Behavioral and Learning Problems.* Roseville, California: Prima Health, 2000.

Seroussi, Karyn. *Unraveling the Mystery of Autism and Pervasive Developmental Disorder.* New York: Simon & Schuster, 2000.

Shaw, William, Ph.D. *Biological Treatments for Autism and PPD.* Overland Park, Kansas: Great Plains Laboratory, 1998.

Williams, Donna. *Nobody Nowhere: The Extraordinary Autobiography of an Autistic.* New York: Times Books, 1992.

Vaccination

Chaitow, Leon. *Vaccination and Immunisation: Dangers, Delusions and Alternatives (What Every Parent Should Know).* Saffron Walden, Essex, England: C. W. Daniel, 1987.

Golden, Isaac. *Vaccination? A Review of Risks and Alternatives,* 5th Ed. Daylesford, Victoria, Australia: Isaac Golden, 1998.

Neustaedter, Randall. *The Vaccine Guide: Making an Informed Choice.* Berkeley, California: North Atlantic Books, 1996.

Smith, Lendon H. *The Infant Survival Guide: Protecting Your Baby from the Dangers of Crib Death, Vaccines and Other Environmental Hazards.* Petaluma, California: Smart Publications, 2000.

Vaccination Roulette. Bangalow, New South Wales, Australia: Australian Vaccination Network (AVN), 1998.

Endnotes

1 What Is Autism?

1. Karyn Seroussi, *Unraveling the Mystery of Autism and Pervasive Developmental Disorder*, New York: Simon & Schuster, 2000, 192.

2. American Psychiatric Association, *DSM-IV-TR (Diagnostic and Statistical Manual of Mental Disorders, 4th Edition, Text Revision)*, Washington, D. C.: American Psychiatric Association, 2000: 75.

3. Dr. Simon Baron-Cohen and Dr. Patrick Bolton, *Autism: The Facts,* New York: Oxford University Press, 1999: 53–9, 71.

4. Temple Grandin and Margaret M. Scariano, *Emergence: Labeled Autistic*, New York: Warner Books, 1996: 146.

5. Ibid., 70, 105.

6. Ibid., 145.

7. E. H. Cook and B. L. Leventhal, "The serotonin system in autism," *Curr Opin Pediatr* 8:4 (August 1996): 348–54.

8. Donna Williams, *Nobody Nowhere: The Extraordinary Autobiography of an Autistic*, New York: Times Books, 1992: 44.

9. J. R. Bemporad, "Adult recollections of a formerly autistic child," *Journal of Autism and Developmental Disorders* 9 (1979): 179–98.

10. From "The Child That You Do Have," written, produced, and directed by Helga-Liz Haberfellner for the cable television series *The Body: Inside Stories*, produced in association with the Discovery Channel and WorkWeek TV Productions.

11. Ibid.

12. Donna Williams, *Nobody Nowhere: The Extraordinary Autobiography of an Autistic*, New York: Times Books, 1992: 10, 72, 129.

13. "Doctors warn developmental disabilities epidemic from toxins," *LDA (Learning Disabilities Association of America) Newsbriefs* 35:4 (July/August 2000): 3; executive summary from the report by the Greater Boston Physicians for Social Responsibility, *In Harm's Way—Toxic Threats to Child Development*, available at www.igc.org/psr/ihw.htm; for LDA, www.ldanatl.org.

14. Autism Autoimmunity Project, "The causes of autism and the need for immunological research: Excerpts from the autism literature," available on the Internet at //http/libnt2.lib.tcu.edu/staff/lruede/immresearch.html (Autism Autoimmunity Project, www.gti.net/truegrit) "U.S. Officials investigate 'cluster' of autism in New Jersey town," CNN, February 1, 1999.

15. U.S. Department of Health and Human Services, "Mental health: A report of the Surgeon General," Rockville, Maryland: U.S. Department of Health and Human Services, Substance Abuse and Mental Health Services Administration, Center for Mental Health Services, National Institutes of Health, National Institute of Mental Health, 1999.

16. Peter E. Tanguay, M.D. "Pervasive developmental disorders: A 10-year review," *Journal of the American Academy of Child and Adolescent Psychiatry* 39:9 (September 2000), 1079–95.

17. Autism Research Institute, personal communication with Dr. Bernard Rimland, 2001.

18. Vaccine Controversies: "Parents of autistic children blame mercury poisoning," *CQ Research* (August 25, 2000), published by Congressional Quarterly, available at the CQ website (www.cq.com).

19. Autism Research Institute, personal communication with Dr. Bernard Rimland, 2001.

20. Bernard Rimland, Ph.D., in "Defeat Autism Now! (DAN!) Mercury Detoxification Consensus Group Position Paper," San Diego, California: Autism Research Institute, May 2001: 3.

21. Ibid.

22. Autism Research Institute, personal communication with Dr. Bernard Rimland, 2001.

23. Geoffrey Cowley, "Understanding autism," *Newsweek* (July 31, 2000).

24. From "The Child That You Do Have," written, produced, and directed by Helga-Liz Haberfellner for the cable television series *The Body: Inside Stories*, produced in association with the Discovery Channel and WorkWeek TV Productions.

25. Sources: Autism Society of America, "Myths about Autism," available on the Internet at www.autism-society.org; Uta Frith, *Autism: Explaining the Enigma*, Cambridge, Massachusetts: Blackwell, 1989; Charles A. Hart, *A Parent's Guide to Autism: Answers to the Most Common Questions*, New York: Pocket Books, 1993; Geoffrey Cowley, "Understanding autism," *Newsweek* (July 31, 2000).

26. Uta Frith, *Autism: Explaining the Enigma*, Cambridge, Massachusetts: Blackwell, 1989: 186.

27. Ibid., 143, 144.

28. Autism Society of America, "Myths about Autism," available on the Internet at www.autism-society.org.

29. Temple Grandin and Margaret M. Scariano, *Emergence: Labeled Autistic*, New York: Warner Books, 1996, 8–9.

30. Dr. Simon Baron-Cohen and Dr. Patrick Bolton, *Autism: The Facts,* New York: Oxford University Press, 1999: 26.

31. Uta Frith, *Autism: Explaining the Enigma*, Cambridge, Massachusetts: Blackwell, 1989: 35, 68–9.

32. *Taber's Cyclopedic Medical Dictionary*, 19th ed., Philadelphia, Pennsylvania: F. A. Davis Company, 2001.

33. Geoffrey Cowley, "Understanding Autism," *Newsweek* (July 31, 2000).

2 Causes and Contributing Factors

34. G. Trottier, et al., "Etiology of infantile autism: A review of recent advances in genetic and neurobiological research," *Journal of Psychiatry and Neuroscience* 24:2 (March 1999): 103–15.

35. Richard Leviton, *The Healthy Living Space*, Charlottesville, Virginia: Hampton Roads, 2001: 2.

36. Ibid., 3.

37. "Doctors warn developmental disabilities epidemic from toxins," *LDA (Learning Disabilities Association of America) Newsbriefs* 35:4 (July/August 2000): 3; executive summary from the report by the Greater Boston Physicians for Social Responsibility, *In Harm's Way—Toxic Threats to Child Development,* available at www.igc.org/psr/ihw.htm; for LDA, www.ldanatl.org.

38. Lynne Cannon, "The Environment and Learning Disabilities," *LDA Newsbriefs* 35:4 (July/August 2000): 1; for LDA, www.ldanatl.org.

39. Ibid.

40. "Doctors warn developmental disabilities epidemic from toxins," *LDA Newsbriefs* 35:4 (July/August 2000): 3–5; executive summary from the report by the Greater Boston Physicians for Social Responsibility, *In Harm's Way—Toxic Threats to Child Development,* available at www.igc.org/psr/ihw.htm; for LDA, www.ldanatl.org.

41. Philip J. Landrigan, *Environmental Neurotoxicology,* Washington, DC: National Academy Press, 1992: 2; cited in Richard Leviton, *The Healthy Living Space,* Charlottesville, Virginia: Hampton Roads, 2001: 13.

42. "Doctors warn developmental disabilities epidemic from toxins," *LDA (Learning Disabilities Association of America) Newsbriefs* 35:4 (July/August 2000): 3–5; executive summary from the report by the Greater Boston Physicians for Social Responsibility, *In Harm's Way—Toxic Threats to Child Development,* available at www.igc.org/psr/ihw.htm; for LDA, www.ldanatl.org.

43. "The Holistic Physician—Autism," *Alternative Medicine Digest* 14 (September 1996): 20.

44. Lawrence Lavine, "Osteopathic and alternative medicine aspects of autistic spectrum disorders," article on the Internet (available at trainland.tripod.com/lawrencelavine.htm).

45. "Elevated serotonin levels in autism: Association with the major histocompatibility complex," *Neuropsychobiology* 34:2 (1996): 72–5.

46. V. K. Singh, "Immunotherapy for brain diseases and mental illnesses," *Progress in Drug Research* 47 (1997): 129–46.

47. Laura J. Ruede, M.L.S., "Autism: An immunological per-

spective," available on the Internet at www.gti.net/truegrit (Autism Autoimmunity Project).

48. Uta Frith, *Autism: Explaining the Enigma*, Cambridge, Massachusetts: Blackwell, 1989: 79–80.

49. A. J. Wakefield, et al., "Ileal-lymphoid-nodular hyperplasia, non-specific colitis, and pervasive developmental disorder in children," *Lancet* 351 (February 28, 1998): 637–41.

50. Andrew J. Wakefield, "Testimony to the Congressional Oversight Committee on Government Reform, available on the Internet at
www.house.gov/reform/hearings/healthcare/01.04.25/wakefield.htm.

51. Bernard Rimland, Ph.D., Editor's Column: "Candida-Caused Autism?" *Autism Research Review International* 2:2 (1988).

52. Ibid.

53. Personal communication, 2001.

54. Mary Callahan, R.N., Guest Editorial: "Autism and allergies: To the parents of kids like Tony," *Autism Research Review International* 3:2 (1989).

55. Ibid.

56. Donna Calvera, "Angela Is Coming Home," in William H. Philpott, M.D., *Brain Allergies*, New Canaan, Connecticut: Keats, 1980.

57. Paul Shattock, "Urinary peptides and associated metabolites in the urine of people with autism spectrum disorders," syllabus material for the main DAN! lecture at the DAN! (Defeat Autism Now!) 2000 Conference, in the conference booklet: 79–83; published by the Autism Research Institute in San Diego, California (fax: 619-563-6840 or website: www.autism.com/ari). "New evidence points to opioids," *Autism Research Review International* 5:4 (1991). A. J. Wakefield, et al., "Ileal-lymphoid-nodular hyperplasia, non-specific colitis, and pervasive developmental disorder in children," *Lancet* 351 (February 28, 1998): 637–41.

58. "New evidence points to opioids," *Autism Research Review International* 5:4 (1991).

59. "New evidence points to opioids," *Autism Research Review International* 5:4 (1991). "Long-term success reported with diet restricting gluten, casein," *Autism Research Review International* 9:4 (1995).

60. Karyn Seroussi, *Unraveling the Mystery of Autism and Pervasive Developmental Disorder*, New York: Simon & Schuster, 2000: 229–30.

61. "Long-term success reported with diet restricting gluten, casein," *Autism Research Review International* 9:4 (1995).

62. Bernard Rimland, Ph.D., "The Feingold diet: An assessment of the reviews by Marttes, by Kavale and Forness and others," *Journal of Learning Disabilities* 16:6 (June/July 1983): 331. (Available from the Autism Research Institute, Publication #51.)

63. Katherine S. Rowe and Kenneth J. Rowe, "Synthetic food coloring and behavior: A dose response effect in a double-blind, placebo-controlled, repeated-measures study," *Journal of Pediatrics* (November 1994): 691–8, in "Color me hyperactive," *Autism Research Review International* 9:2 (1995).

64. Hyman J. Roberts, "Reactions attributed to aspartame containing products: 551 cases," *Natural Food & Farming* (March 1992): 23–8.

65. Information at www.feingold.org/symptoms-main.html

66. Bernard Rimland, Ph.D., "The Feingold diet: An assessment of the reviews by Marttes, by Kavale and Forness and others," *Journal of Learning Disabilities* 16:6 (June/July 1983): 331. (Available from the Autism Research Institute, Publication #51.)

67. Ibid.

68. Claudio Galli and Artemis P. Simopoulos, ed., *Dietary W3 and W6 Fatty Acids: Biological Effects and Nutritional Essentiality*, New York: Kluwer/Plenum, 1989. Claudio Galli and Artemis P. Simopoulos, *Effects of Fatty Acids and Lipids in Health and Disease,* New York: S. Karger, 1994. Joseph Mercola, "Where's the Real Beef?" available on the Internet at www.mercola.com/beef/main.htm.

69. Presenter statement by Andrew Stoll, M.D., in the DAN! (Defeat Autism Now!) 2000 Conference booklet: 8; published by the Autism Research Institute in San Diego, California (fax: 619-563-6840 or website: www.autism.com/ari).

70. M. A. Crawford, A. G. Hassam, and P. A. Stevens, "Essential fatty acid requirements in pregnancy and lactation with special reference to brain development," *Prog Lipid Res* 20 (1981): 31–40.

71. "Healing mood disorders with essential fatty acids," *Doctors' Prescription for Healthy Living* 4:6, 1.

72. Patricia Kane, Ph.D., "Reversing Autism with Nutrition," *Alternative Medicine Digest* 19 (August/September 1997): 42.

73. Ibid.

74. Bernard Rimland, Ph.D., "Form letter regarding high dosage vitamin B_6 and magnesium therapy for autism and related disorders," revised April 1998. (Available from the Autism Research Institute, Publication #39G.)

75. ———"The use of megavitamin B_6 and magnesium in the treatment of autistic children and adults," in E. Schopler and G. Mesibov, eds., *Neurobiological Issues in Autism*, New York: Plenum, 1987: 389–405. (Available from the Autism Research Institute, Publication #81.)

76. Ibid.

77. ——— "The most airtight study in psychiatry? Vitamin B_6 in autism," *Autism Research Review International* 14:3 (2000).

78. ——— "Form letter regarding high dosage vitamin B_6 and magnesium therapy for autism and related disorders," revised April 1998. (Available from the Autism Research Institute, Publication #39G.)

79. ——— "Dimethyglycine (DMG), a nontoxic metabolite, and autism," *Autism Research Review International* 4:2 (1990).

80. Ibid.

81. ——— "Form letter regarding high dosage vitamin B_6 and magnesium therapy for autism and related disorders," revised April 1998. (Available from the Autism Research Institute, Publication #39G.)

82. ——— "The use of megavitamin B_6 and magnesium in the treatment of autistic children and adults," in E. Schopler and G. Mesibov, eds., *Neurobiological Issues in Autism*, New York: Plenum, 1987: 389–405. (Available from the Autism Research Institute, Publication #81.)

83. Mary Megson, M.D., "Is autism a G-alpha protein defect reversible with natural vitamin A?" *Medical Hypotheses* 54:6 (2000): 979–83.

84. ——— "Is autism a G-alpha protein defect reversible with natural vitamin A?" *Medical Hypotheses* 54:6 (2000): 980.

85. ——— "Is autism a G-alpha protein defect reversible with natural vitamin A?" *Medical Hypotheses* 54:6 (2000): 981.

86. M. C. Dolske, et al., "A preliminary trial of ascorbic acid as supplemental therapy for autism," *Prog Neuropsychopharmacol Biol* Psychiatry 17:5 (September 1993): 765–74.

87. Lelland C. Tolbert, "Ascorbic acid: Therapeutic trial in autism," presentation at the Autism Society of America annual conference, Indianapolis, Indiana, July 10–13, 1991. Reported in "Ascorbic acid and autism," *Autism Research Review International* 6:1 (1992).

3 The Vaccine and Mercury Controversy

88. Vaccine Adverse Event Reporting System, "VAERS Data," available on the Internet at www.vaers.org/info.htm.

89. Illinois Vaccine Awareness Coalition, "Vaccine Fact Sheet," available on the Internet at www.vaccineawareness.org/information/FactSheet.htm.

90. Ibid.

91. Lisa Reagan, "Show us the science," *Mothering* (March–April 2001): 43.

92. Bernard Rimland, Ph.D., Editor's Notebook: "The Autism Explosion," *Autism Research Review International* 13:2 (1999).

93. Tim O'Shea, D. C., "Autism and Vaccine," available on the Internet at www.chiroweb.com/archives/18/25/02.html.

94. Ibid.

95. Tinus Smits, "The Post-Vaccination Syndrome: Basic Description," available on the Internet at www.tinussmits.com/english/.

96. Available on the National Vaccine Information Center website at www.909shot.com/NVICSpecialReport.htm.

97. Ibid.

98. Tim O'Shea, D. C., "Autism and Mercury: The San Diego Conference," report on the DAN! 2000 Conference, September 15, 2000, San Diego, California, available on the Internet at www.chiroweb.com/archives/19/05/02.html.

99. Andrew J. Wakefield, "Testimony to the Congressional Oversight Committee on Government Reform," available on the Internet at www.house.gov/reform/hearings/healthcare/01.04.25/wakefield.htm.

100. "Adverse events associated with childhood vaccines," report by the Institute of Medicine, 1994, cited in "Hepatitis B disease and vaccine facts," available at the National Vaccine Information Center website: www.909shot.com/hepBfacts.htm.

101. Lisa Reagan, "Show us the science," *Mothering* (March–April 2001): 43.

102. Ibid., 52.

103. "Vaccine safety group endorses government action to eliminate mercury in childhood vaccines and roll back hepatitis B vaccination for most newborn infants," NVIC press release (July 8, 1999), available on the Internet at www.909shot.com/thimersolpr.htm.

104. Lisa Suhay, "Delay urged for vaccine with a trace of mercury," *New York Times* (July 18, 1999). NVIC Special Report, available on the Internet at www.909shot.com/NVICSpecialReport.htm.

105. Vaccine Controversies: "Parents of autistic children blame mercury poisoning," *CQ Research* (August 25, 2000): 661, published by Congressional Quarterly, available at the CQ website (www.cq.com).

106. NVIC Special Report, available on the Internet at www.909shot.com/NVICSpecialReport.htm.

107. Dawn Winkler, "Vaccine Ingredients," available on the Internet at www.tetrahedron.org/articles/vaccine_awareness/ingredients.html.

108. "Five drug makers use material with possible mad cow link," *New York Times* (February 8, 2001): Business Day.

109. Data available at www.fda.gov/oc/opacom/hottopics/bse.html.

110. VAERS Statistics, compiled by the Illinois Vaccine Awareness Coalition, available on the Internet at www.vaccineawareness.org/information/VAERS_statistics.htm.

111. VAERS Data, available on the Internet at www.vaers.org/ info.htm

112. Lisa Reagan, "Show us the science," *Mothering* (March–April 2001): 47–8.

113. Tinus Smits, "The Post-Vaccination Syndrome: Prevention," available on the Internet at www.tinussmits.com/english/

114. Dietrich Klinghardt, M.D., Ph.D., "Amalgam/mercury detox as a treatment for chronic viral, bacterial, and fungal illnesses," lecture presented at the Annual Meeting of the International and

American Academy of Clinical Nutrition, San Diego, California, September 1996.

115. W. M. Egan, "Thimerosal in vaccines," presentation to the FDA (September 14, 1999), cited in Sallie Bernard, et al., "Autism: a novel form of mercury poisoning," available from ARC Research, 14 Commerce Drive, Cranford, New Jersey 07901 (tel: 908-276-6300); available on the Internet at www.mercola.com/2000/oct/1/autism_mercury.htm.

116. Vaccine Controversies: "Parents of autistic children blame mercury poisoning," *CQ Research* (August 25, 2000): 660, published by *Congressional Quarterly*, available at the CQ website (www.cq.com).

117. "Doctors warn developmental disabilities epidemic from toxins," *LDA (Learning Disabilities Association of America) Newsbriefs* 35:4 (July/August 2000): 3–5; executive summary from the report by the Greater Boston Physicians for Social Responsibility, *In Harm's Way—Toxic Threats to Child Development*, available at www.igc.org/psr/ihw.htm; for LDA, www.ldanatl.org.

118. David Poulson, "Danger from mercury higher than thought," *San Francisco Chronicle* (March 3, 2001).

119. Sallie Bernard, et al., "Autism: a novel form of mercury poisoning," available from ARC Research, 14 Commerce Drive, Cranford, New Jersey 07901 (tel: 908-276-6300); available on the Internet at www.mercola.com/2000/oct/1/autism_mercury.htm.

120. Lisa Reagan, "What about mercury?," *Mothering* (March–April 2001): 54–5.

121. "Mercury in medicine—are we taking unnecessary risks?" *DAMS (Dental Amalgam Mercury Syndrome)* 13 (Spring/Summer 2000): 1.

122. Rosie Waterhouse, "Autism Linked to Mercury Vaccine," UK Times, available on the Internet at www.mercola.com/2001/jun/13/autism_mercury.htm

123. Press release from PROVE (Parents Requesting Open Vaccine Education), available on the Internet at www.vaccineinfo.net/autismHg.htm or www.mercola.com/2001/ oct/31/mercury_lawsuit.htm.

124. Ibid.

125. "Vaccines under fire," *International DAMS (Dental Amalgam Mercury Syndrome)Newsletter* (March 2000): 3.

4 Targeted Therapeutic Nutrition and Heavy-Metal Detoxification

126. William Shaw, Ph.D., *Biological Treatments for Autism and PPD*, Overland Park, Kansas: Great Plains Laboratory, 1998: 45.

127. S. Klein, "Glutamine: an essential nonessential amino acid for the gut," *Gastroenterology* 99:1 (1990): 279–81.

128. G.B.J. Glass and B.L. Slomiany, "Derangements of biosynthesis, production and secretion of mucus in gastrointestinal injury and disease," *Adv Exp Med Biol* 89 (1976): 311–47. A. Herp et al., "Biochemistry and lectin binding properties of mammalian salivary mucous glycoproteins," *Adv Exp Med Biol* 228 (1988): 395–435.

129. S. Pullman-Mooar et al., "Alteration of the cellular fatty acid profile and the production of eicosanoids in human monocytes by gamma-linolenic acid," *Arthritis and Rheumatism* 33:10 (1990): 1526–33. G. Tate et al., "Suppression of acute and chronic inflammation by dietary gamma linolenic acid," *Journal of Rheumatology* 16:6 (1989): 729–34. D.F. Horrobin, "Interactions between n-3 and n-6 essential fatty acids (EFAs) in the regulation of cardiovascular disorders and inflammation," *Prostaglandins Leukotrienes and Essential Fatty Acids* 44 (1991): 127–31. D.E. Barre and B.J. Holub, "The effect of borage oil consumption on human plasma lipid levels and the phosphatidylcholine and cholesterol ester composition of high density lipoprotein," *Nutrition Research* 12 (1992): 1181–94.

130. T. Takemoto et al., "Practical usage of gamma-oryzanol on chronic gastritis," *Shinyaku to Rinsho* 25:5 (1976): 3. K. Maruyama et al., "Usefulness of Hi-Z fine granules (gamma-oryzanol) for the treatment of indefinite digestive tract complaints," *Shinyaku to Rinsho* 25:8 (1976): 3.

131. David L. Hoffman, M.N.I.M.H., *The New Holistic Herbal*, Boston, Massachusetts: Element Books, 1990: 233.

132. Kerry Bone, "Globe Artichoke: Therapeutic and Medicinal Properties," *Nutrition and Healing* (July 1998): 3–4. Melvyn R. Werbach, M.D., and Michael T. Murray, N.D., *Botanical Influences*

on Illness: A Sourcebook of Clinical Research. New Canaan, Connecticut: Keats Publishing, 1988: 28

5 NAET: Allergy-Related Autism

133. Adapted from Devi S. Nambudripad, D.C., L.Ac., R.N., Ph.D., *Say Goodbye to Allergy-Related Autism,* Buena Park, California: Delta Publishing, 1999: 32–47. Devi S. Nambudripad, D.C., L.Ac., R.N., Ph.D., *Say Goodbye to Illness,* New & Revised ed., Buena Park, California: Delta Publishing, 1999: 296.

134. Nambudripad, *Illness,* xxii.

135. Personal communication with Dr. Nambudripad, 2001. Richard Leviton, "The Allergy-Free Body," *Alternative Medicine Digest* 6 (April 1995): 13.

136. Nambudripad, *Illness,* xxiii.

137. ——— *Autism,* vii.

138. ——— *Illness,* 147–148.

139. ——— *Autism,* 201.

140. Ibid., 28–31.

141. Ibid., 200.

142. Ibid.

143. Richard Leviton, "The Allergy-Free Body," *Alternative Medicine Digest* 6 (April 1995): 8.

144. Nambudripad, *Autism,* 234–236.

145. Personal communication with Dr. Nambudripad, 2001. Nambudripad, *Autism,* 221–224.

146. Nambudripad, *Autism,* 237–244.

6 Biochemical Therapy and a Landmark Discovery

147. William J. Walsh, Ph.D. Proceedings of the American Psychiatric Association, May 2001, New Orleans, Louisiana.

148. Ibid.

149. ——— "The critical role of nutrients in severe mental symptoms," available on the Internet (www.alternativemental-health.com/articles/article-pffeiffer.htm).

150. ——— "Biochemical treatment: medicines for the next century," *NOHA (Nutrition for Optimal Health Association) News* 16:3 (Summer 1991), available on the HRIPTC Website

(www.hriptc.org/nextcentury.htm). Richard Leviton, "Schizophrenia: Healing the Divided Self with Nutrients," *Alternative Medicine* 24 (June/July 1998): 44–46.

151. ——— "The critical role of nutrients in severe mental symptoms," available on the Internet (www.alternativemental-health.com/articles/article-pffeiffer.htm).

152. Donna Williams, *Nobody Nowhere: The Extraordinary Autobiography of an Autistic*, New York: Times Books, 1992: 202.

153. William J. Walsh, Ph.D., "Biochemical treatment: medicines for the next century," *NOHA (Nutrition for Optimal Health Association) News* 16:3 (Summer 1991), available on the HRIPTC Website (www.hriptc.org/nextcentury.htm). William J. Walsh, Ph.D., "The critical role of nutrients in severe mental symptoms," available on the Internet (www.alternativementalhealth.com/articles/article-pffeiffer.htm).

7 Homeopathy: Constitutional Treatment, Vaccine Clearing, and an Alternative to Vaccines

154. Miranda Castro, R.S.Hom., *The Complete Homeopathy Handbook*, New York: St. Martin's Press, 1990: 3–5. Anne Woodham and David Peters, M.D., *Encyclopedia of Healing Therapies*, New York: Dorling Kindersley, 1997: 126.

155. Judyth Reichenberg-Ullman, N.D., M.S.W., and Robert Ullman, N.D., *Ritalin-Free Kids: Safe and Effective Homeopathic Medicine for ADHD, and Other Behavioral and Learning Problems,* Roseville, California: Prima Health, 2000: 95.

156. Ibid., 95–96.

157. Personal communication, 2001. Judyth Reichenberg-Ullman, N.D., M.S.W., and Robert Ullman, N.D., *Ritalin-Free Kids: Safe and Effective Homeopathic Medicine for ADHD, and Other Behavioral and Learning Problems,* Roseville, California: Prima Health, 2000: 218–219.

158. *R.-F. Kids,* 90.

159. Ibid., 86.

160. Ibid., 83.

161. Ibid., 210.

162. Published in *Similia,* Journal of the AHA 7:1 (1994). Available at www.homeopathyoz.org.

163. Francisco X. Eizayaga, M.D., "Prevention of Infectious Diseases," in Richard E. Hiltner, M.D., D.Ht., and Francisco X. Eizayaga, M.D. "Homeopathy and Immunizations," self-published, available through Dr. Hiltner (see address in appendix B: Resources).

164. Ibid.

165. See *Homeopathic Guide—Vaccination Damage*, by Carola Lage-Roy and Ravi Roy (Murnau, Germany: Lage and Roy, 1976).

166. For more about Dr. Philip Incao's work, see www.compwellness.com/mp/incaop.htm or www.garynull.com/Documents/niin/Philip_Incao.htm

167. Philip Incao, M.D., "Supporting Children's Health," *Alternative Medicine Digest* 19 August/September 1997): 54.

168. Ibid., 55.

169. William Cookson and Miriam Moffatt, "Asthma: An epidemic in the absence of infection?" *Science* 275 (January 3, 1997): 41–42.

170. Tove Ronne, "Measles virus infection without rash in childhood is related to disease in adult life," *Lancet* 1:8419 (January 5, 1985): 1–5.

171. N. P. Thompson, et al., "Is measles vaccination a risk factor for inflammatory bowel disease?" *Lancet* 1:8419 (January 5, 1985): 1–5.

172. Philip Incao, M.D., "Supporting Children's Health," *Alternative Medicine Digest* 19 August/September 1997): 59.

173. Ibid.,57.

174. Ibid.,59.

175. Ibid., 54, 56.

8 Cranial Osteopathy: The Role of Birth Trauma in Autism

176. H. I. Magoun, D.O., *Osteopathy in the Cranial Field*, 3d Ed., Kirksville, MO: Journal Printing Company, 1976: 1.

177. "What Is Osteopathy?" available at the Cranial Academy Website (www.cranialacademy.org/whatis.html).

178. "Common Problems," available at the Cranial Academy Website (www.cranialacademy.org/cmpr.html).

179. Lawrence Lavine, "Osteopathic and alternative medicine aspects of autistic spectrum disorders," article on the Internet (avail-

able at trainland.tripod.com/lawrencelavine.htm).

180. E. Courchesne, "Neuroanatomical systems involved in infantile autism: The implications of cerebellar abnormalities," In G. Dawson, *Autism: Nature, Diagnosis, and Treatment,* New York: Guilford Press, 1989: 180–143.

181. Lawrence Lavine, "Osteopathic and alternative medicine aspects of autistic spectrum disorders," article on the Internet (available at trainland.tripod.com/lawrencelavine.htm).

182. Ibid.

9 Soma Therapies: Structural, Functional, and Emotional Release

183. "CranioSacral Therapy," available at the Upledger Institute Website www.upledger.com/therapies/cst.htm.

184. "What is Osteopathy?" available at the Cranial Academy Website www.cranialacademy.org/whatis.html.

185. "CranioSacral Therapy," available at the Upledger Institute Website www.upledger.com/therapies/cst.htm.

186. Sources: Informational materials of Soma Therapy Centre. Richard Leviton, "Reversing Autism and Depression with Bodywork," *Alternative Medicine* 24 (June/July 1998): 36–41.

187. Richard Leviton, "Reversing Autism and Depression with Bodywork," *Alternative Medicine* 24 (June/July 1998): 36–41.

188. Ibid., 39.

10 The Tomatis Method: Listening and Autism

189. From "The Child That You Do Have," written, produced, and directed by Helga-Liz Haberfellner for the cable television series *The Body: Inside Stories,* produced in association with the Discovery Channel and WorkWeek TV Productions. Personal communication with Paul Madaule, 2001.

190. Paul Madaule, *When Listening Comes Alive: A Guide to Effective Learning and Communication,* Norval, Ontario, Canada: Moulin, 1994: 35–36.

191. Internet information, available at www.tomatis. com/English/Articles/autism.htm. Personal communication with Paul Madaule, 2001.

192. Nicholas Regush, "The Listening Cure," *Equinox* (April/May 1997): 72–74.

193. From "The Child That You Do Have," written, produced, and directed by Helga-Liz Haberfellner for the cable television series *The Body: Inside Stories*, produced in association with the Discovery Channel and WorkWeek TV Productions.

194. Ibid., Pierre Sollier, M.F.C.C., "Ask the Physician: Healing with Music," *Alternative Medicine* 25 (August/September 1998): 34–38.

195. Paul Madaule, *When Listening Comes Alive: A Guide to Effective Learning and Communication*, Norval, Ontario, Canada: Moulin, 1994: 41–42.

196. From "The Child That You Do Have," written, produced, and directed by Helga-Liz Haberfellner for the cable television series *The Body: Inside Stories*, produced in association with the Discovery Channel and WorkWeek TV Productions. Pierre Sollier, M.F.C.C., "Ask the Physician: Healing with Music," *Alternative Medicine* 25 (August/September 1998): 34–38.

197. Paul Madaule, *When Listening Comes Alive: A Guide to Effective Learning and Communication*, Norval, Ontario, Canada: Moulin, 1994: 65–66.

198. Ibid., 66.

199. From "The Child That You Do Have," written, produced, and directed by Helga-Liz Haberfellner for the cable television series *The Body: Inside Stories*, produced in association with the Discovery Channel and WorkWeek TV Productions.

200. Internet information, available at www.aitresources.com and www.thedaviscenter.com/therapies/t-ait.html.

11 Neural Therapy, Toxic Clearing, and Family Systems Therapy: The Levels of Healing

201. Richard Leviton, "Migraines, Seizures, and Mercury Toxicity," *Alternative Medicine Digest* 21 (December 1997/January 1998): 61.

Index

About the Author

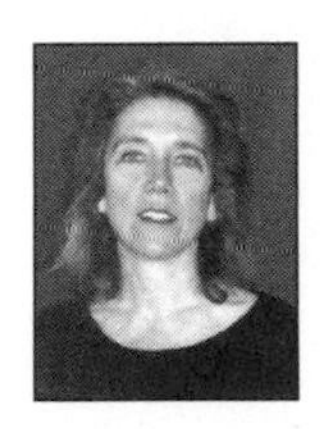

Stephanie Marohn has been writing since she was a child. Her adult writing background is extensive in both journalism and nonfiction trade books. In addition to *Natural Medicine First Aid Remedies* and the six books in the Healthy Mind Series *(The Natural Medicine Guide to Autism, The Natural Medicine Guide to Depression, The Natural Medicine Guide to Bipolar Depression, The Natural Medicine Guide to Addiction, The Natural Medicine Guide to Anxiety,* and *The Natural Medicine Guide to Schizophrenia)*, she has published more than thirty articles in magazines and newspapers, written two novels and a feature film screenplay, and has had her work included in poetry, prayer, and travel writing anthologies.

Originally from Philadelphia, she has been a resident of the San Francisco Bay Area for over twenty years, and currently lives in Sonoma Country, north of the city.

Please visit www.stephaniemarohn.com for more information.

Hampton Roads Publishing Company

. . . for the evolving human spirit

Hampton Roads Publishing Company
publishes books on a variety of subjects,
including metaphysics, health, integrative medicine,
visionary fiction, and other related topics.

For a copy of our latest catalog, call toll-free
800-766-8009, or send your name and address to:

Hampton Roads Publishing Company, Inc.
1125 Stoney Ridge Road
Charlottesville, VA 22902

e-mail: hrpc@hrpub.com
www.hrpub.com